Happy Feet, Healthy Food

Your Child's First Journal of
Exercise and Healthy Eating

Carol Goodrow

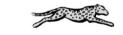

BREAKAWAY BOOKS
HALCOTTSVILLE, NEW YORK
2004

Happy Feet, Healthy Food: Your Child's First Journal of Exercise and Healthy Eating

Copyright 2004 by Carol Goodrow

ISBN: 1-891369-46-6
Library of Congress Control Number: 2003116286

PRINTED IN CHINA

Published by Breakaway Books
P. O. Box 24
Halcottsville, NY 12438
(800) 548-4348
www.breakawaybooks.com

FIRST EDITION

DEDICATION
Reason to Dedicate "Love" If a child takes a book to heart it may change that child's life.

This book is dedicated to all children who love physical activity and healthy eating, including my many schoolchildren for the past 7 years.

It's also dedicated to the many children who have yet to discover the joys of exercise and nutritious food in hopes that this book will inspire and enrich their lives.

ACKNOWLEDGEMENTS
Reason to Acknowledge "More Love" This is my chance to thank and send love to all the people who directly helped make this book happen.

First, I'd like to thank Ambrose (Amby) Burfoot, my editor from Runner's World Magazine, for urging me to write this book. It was Amby's astute sense of mission that made me understand the importance of encouraging our young people to embrace healthy lifestyles. Furthermore, without Amby's continued close attention to my work I may never have acquired the confidence needed to create this book.

Next, I'd like to thank Garth Battista, my publisher, who took a chance with me and said, "Yes," to this project. I'd also like to thank three very encouraging friends: Diane Hutton, Lori Adams, and Bob Mills who always found value in my creativity, my children Josie and Keith, who have put up with a lifetime of my creative endeavors, my mother for taking me to the library when I was young, my classroom aide, Fran Mloganoski, who has started running (in her sixties), my 14 week-old puppy dog Captain "Yellow" Midnight for giving the book a little pep, and my librarian, Linda Gallic for help with the research.

Finally, I'd like to thank my non-running husband, Kevin, for trekking out with me every weekend to the hills of Wells State Park and for supporting me in every way imaginable.

FOREWORD
by Amby Burfoot

When I was younger, I thought Albert Einstein was the world's only real genius and his famous equation $E=MC^2$, was the proof of his genius. Now I am older and wiser, and I realize genius takes many forms.

The book in your hands is a work of genius. I say this with certainty because this is the first book to recognize that we must begin to teach our kids about good health and nutrition at a young age. When we wait longer, as we have for too long, we end up raising kids who are overweight and out-of-shape, as newspapers now tell us almost every morning. Others will soon wake up and produce more books and videos to encourage kids' fitness, but this will be difficult for anyone else to improve upon it.

This book couldn't have come into existence without the genius of Carol Goodrow. I have known Carol for a half-dozen years, and I have been continually amazed at her energy, intelligence, and, most important of all, her good heart. She has astounded me with the boundless enthusiasm she has poured into her Web site, www.kidsrunning.com. It is a fun and info-packed place for youngsters to learn about running and good health.

This book is all that, and more. Part of Carol's genius is the way she integrates fitness with the traditional school subjects. When your kids use this book, often with you at their side, they won't just get healthier. They'll also practice basic counting skills, and write short stories about food, exercise, and the outside environment.

A number of research studies have shown that aerobic exercise floods the brain with oxygen, unlocking its creativity. Carol uses this simple, scientific fact to help you raise a healthier and faster learning child. You could hardly ask for more.

I hope you'll open this book often with your child. You'll both be glad you did. And you'll continue to see the benefits for many years to come-perhaps even a lifetime.

Amby Burfoot, Executive Editor, RUNNER'S WORLD Magazine
Boston Marathon Winner, 1968

INTRODUCTION
by Carol Goodrow

Writing HAPPY FEET, HEALTHY FOOD has been a lot of fun for me. It's pretty cool to put creative ideas into a book, knowing that someday you'll see the book in the hands of a child.

The book started out as a simple diary for children to record their physical activity and healthy eating, then it began to fill up with mini-stories of the experiences I've had that changed my life: stories of running with my schoolchildren on a woodsy trail, choosing fruit instead of candy to prevent disease, exercising to strengthen my heart, eating vegetables to become lean, cycling to raise money to find a cure for cancer, and playing with my puppy outdoors for some healthy fun.

I hope that as you turn the pages of my book, you decide to join in the fun by trying the activities and the healthy food. And when you do, please invite your families to join you. Feel free to invent some activities of your own. Then record your thoughts and adventures, thus turning the book into the mini-stories of your life.

Stay happy, get lean and fit, keep your feet moving, pack a healthy snack for school, and have fun with HAPPY FEET, HEALTHY FOOD.

USING THE JOURNAL PAGES

Reason to Journal "Memories" Your journal pages are like a scrapbook. They'll turn this book into the story of your life.

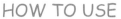

HOW TO USE

The journal pages have 4 parts: a physical activity log, a time tracker, a healthy food 9-square, and a writer & artist's corner. The more you record, the more complete your "story" will be.

WRITING AND ART TOOLS

Pencils and colored pencils are the recommended tools. Other art supplies can be used but they may bleed through to the other side of the page.

PHYSICAL ACTIVITY LOG

Use this log to fill in your physical activities each day. Here are some example

Heidi, age 6

Monday:	RUN.
Tuesday:	PLAY SOCCER.

Alexander, age 10

Monday:	Ran at the high school track with Mom and Dad. Started RAINING right after our run.
Tuesday:	Kicked the soccer ball around down at the field with Sara at recess. Ran in the back yard after school.

Diane, age 13

Monday:	Ran 2 miles at running club (16 minutes). Did 10 push-ups. Went for a walk up Cedar Street after supper with the family.
Tuesday:	Walked at recess with Mia and Susie. Soccer practice after school. Did drills, scored 2 goals, stretched for 10 minutes.

USING THE JOURNAL PAGES (continued)

TIME TRACKER (optional)

Use this time grid to keep track of every 10 minutes of exercise. Simply fill in the squares. Use a watch, timer, or clock, when you can. Find out how long your recess and gym classes are. Then fill in 2 squares for 20 minutes, or 3 squares for 30 minutes.

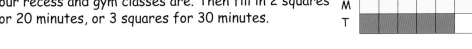

HEALTHY FOOD 9-SQUARE

Make it your goal to ALWAYS have this grid completed by the end of each week. Since you should be eating healthy foods all the time, you should easily reach this goal.

Use stickers, smilies, WOW's, X's, hearts, stars, A+'s, apples, rainbows, or any creative method you can think of to record fruits, vegetables, and any food mentioned in this book. You can write the names of the foods in the squares or you may wish to create abbreviations or use the beginning letter of the food (like "pap" or "p" for papaya).

WRITER & ARTIST'S CORNER

Each page has a little spot for creativity. This is the place where you can really do your own thing. Anything goes ! Here are three examples.

A Motto   Evaluation and Goal   Your Pick

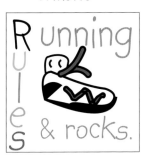

Running
R
U
l
e
S
& rocks.

Did great at skating this week. Ride more next week.

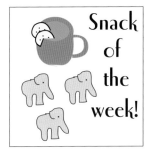

Snack of the week!

RUN

REASON TO RUN "Heat" You'll burn calories.

FUN FEET
Run
Play chase with your puppy.

Chase butterflies.

Play tag with your friends.

Chase your shadow.

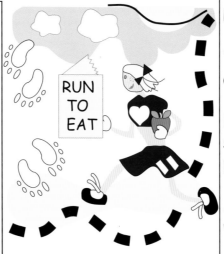

RUN TO EAT

LEAN & FIT KIDS
run and eat fruit.

PACK-A-SNACK
Apples
Whole fresh apple

Half-apple spread with peanut butter

Apple slices with cinnamon

Apples with salads

Apples in muffins

GOOD STUFF
Apples
-Lots of vitamin C to help your skin heal

-Fiber

-Low calories

- Wash before you eat.

Monday's date _____

PHYSICAL ACTIVITY LOG

Record your physical activity for each day of the week. Older kids, record all of your physical activity. (Ex: Ran a mile with Dad. Rode my bike a block to Drew's house.) Younger kids, write at least one word to indicate your physical activity. (Ex: Soccer)

Monday:

Tuesday:

Wednesday:

Thursday:

Friday:

Saturday:

Sunday:

TIME TRACKER (optional)
Color in a section for every 10 minutes of exercise you have completed each day. Goal: 1 hour of daily exercise.

HEALTHY FOOD 9-SQUARE
Make a smile face or place a sticker for every healthy food, found in this book, that you've eaten this week.

WRITER & ARTIST'S CORNER
Make a sketch or write down thoughts about your exercise or healthy eating this week. Possible topics include: goals, nature, and food.

M
T
W
H
F
S
S

WALK

Reason to Walk   "Lifetime Activity" Walking is an activity for people of all ages.

FUN FEET
Walk

Walk to school.

Walk with your friends.

Walk with your sisters and brothers.

Walk with your parents.

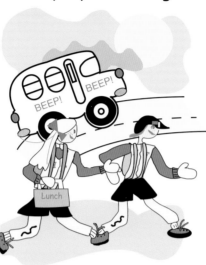

LEAN & FIT KIDS choose walking over riding.

PACK-A-SNACK
Lunchbox
Sandwich Special

Whole-wheat bread (whole grain)

Romaine lettuce (vegetable)

Lean meat (protein)

Low-fat cheese (low-fat dairy)

Thin slices of avocados (fruit/fat)

GOOD STUFF
Lunchbox

-Fresh fruit   -Lean protein

-Low-fat dairy   -Vegetables

-Whole grains   -Water

-Healthy fat

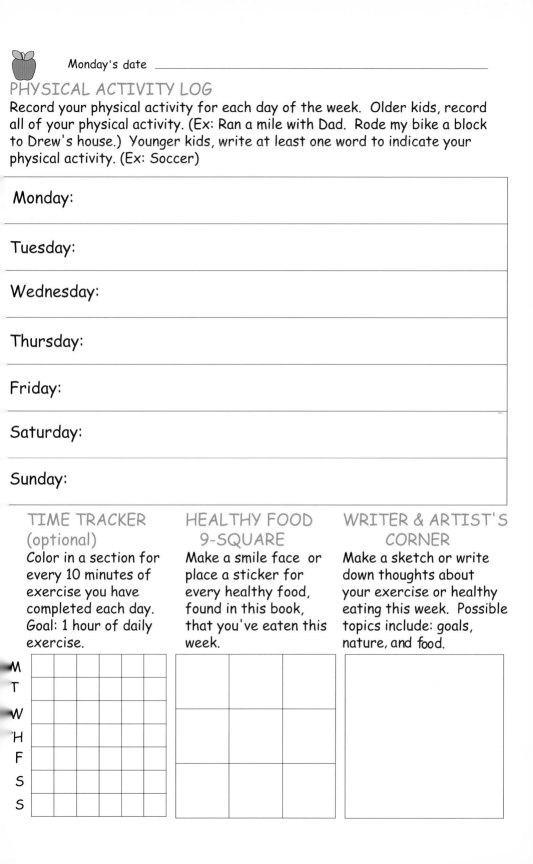

Monday's date _____

PHYSICAL ACTIVITY LOG

Record your physical activity for each day of the week. Older kids, record all of your physical activity. (Ex: Ran a mile with Dad. Rode my bike a block to Drew's house.) Younger kids, write at least one word to indicate your physical activity. (Ex: Soccer)

Monday:

Tuesday:

Wednesday:

Thursday:

Friday:

Saturday:

Sunday:

TIME TRACKER (optional)

Color in a section for every 10 minutes of exercise you have completed each day. Goal: 1 hour of daily exercise.

M
T
W
H
F
S
S

HEALTHY FOOD 9-SQUARE

Make a smile face or place a sticker for every healthy food, found in this book, that you've eaten this week.

WRITER & ARTIST'S CORNER

Make a sketch or write down thoughts about your exercise or healthy eating this week. Possible topics include: goals, nature, and food.

HIKE

Reason to Hike "Strength" You will build strong leg and ankle muscles.

FUN FEET
Hike

Walk in the woods.

Climb a hill or mountain.

Walk on a trail.

Hike with your mom or dad for safety.

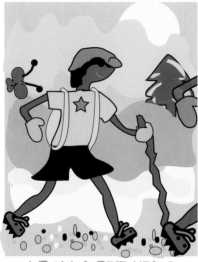

LEAN & FIT KIDS snack while they hike.

PACK-A-SNACK
Trail Mix

Chopped walnuts

Almonds

Sunflower seeds

Dry cereal

Dried fruit

Few chocolate chips or m&m's

GOOD STUFF
Trail Mix

-Nuts and seeds have healthy fat.

-Dried fruit has potassium.

-Cereal has B vitamins.

-Eat small portions of trail mix.

Monday's date _____

PHYSICAL ACTIVITY LOG

Record your physical activity for each day of the week. Older kids, record all of your physical activity. (Ex: Ran a mile with Dad. Rode my bike a block to Drew's house.) Younger kids, write at least one word to indicate your physical activity. (Ex: Soccer)

Monday:

Tuesday:

Wednesday:

Thursday:

Friday:

Saturday:

Sunday:

TIME TRACKER (optional)	HEALTHY FOOD 9-SQUARE	WRITER & ARTIST'S CORNER
Color in a section for every 10 minutes of exercise you have completed each day. Goal: 1 hour of daily exercise.	Make a smile face or place a sticker for every healthy food, found in this book, that you've eaten this week.	Make a sketch or write down thoughts about your exercise or healthy eating this week. Possible topics include: goals, nature, and food.

M
T
W
H
F
S
S

RUN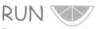

Reason to Run "Awards" If you finish a fun run, you might get a ribbon, trophy, or medal.

FUN FEET
Fun Run
Warm up
by jogging.

Run slowly at
the start.

Pick up the
pace later.

Keep running
until you
cross the
finish line.

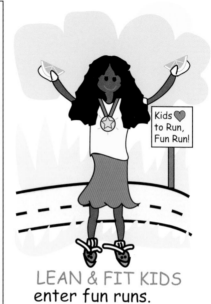

Kids ♥ to Run, Fun Run!

LEAN & FIT KIDS
enter fun runs.

PACK-A-SNACK
Oranges
Eat before,
during, or after
a fun run.

Peel, but leave
the white skin
on the orange.

Eat plain and
in fruit salads.

Drink a small
glass of orange
juice.

GOOD STUFF
Oranges
-Lots of vitamin C

-Quick energy

-Fiber

-Runners often eat oranges at events.

Monday's date _____

PHYSICAL ACTIVITY LOG

Record your physical activity for each day of the week. Older kids, record all of your physical activity. (Ex: Ran a mile with Dad. Rode my bike a block to Drew's house.) Younger kids, write at least one word to indicate your physical activity. (Ex: Soccer)

Monday:

Tuesday:

Wednesday:

Thursday:

Friday:

Saturday:

Sunday:

TIME TRACKER (optional)
Color in a section for every 10 minutes of exercise you have completed each day. Goal: 1 hour of daily exercise.

HEALTHY FOOD 9-SQUARE
Make a smile face or place a sticker for every healthy food, found in this book, that you've eaten this week.

WRITER & ARTIST'S CORNER
Make a sketch or write down thoughts about your exercise or healthy eating this week. Possible topics include: goals, nature, and food.

M
T
W
H
F
S
S

EXERCISE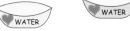

Reason to Exercise "Fun" It's fun for people and dogs to exercise together.

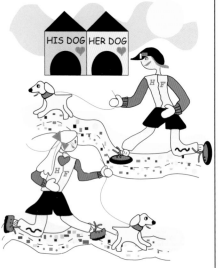

HIS DOG HER DOG

LEAN & FIT KIDS
play with their dogs.

FUN FEET
Exercise
Run with your dog.

Walk your dog.

Play Frisbee with your dog.

Take your dog for a swim.

PACK-A-SNACK
Dog Snacks
Water

Little bits of skinless cooked chicken or turkey breast, no bones

Dog biscuits

Shredded carrots

GOOD STUFF
Dog Snacks
-Dog biscuits for healthy gums

-Chicken for protein

-Water to keep your dog hydrated

-Don't overdo treats or snacks.

Monday's date _____

PHYSICAL ACTIVITY LOG

Record your physical activity for each day of the week. Older kids, record all of your physical activity. (Ex: Ran a mile with Dad. Rode my bike a block to Drew's house.) Younger kids, write at least one word to indicate your physical activity. (Ex: Soccer)

Monday:

Tuesday:

Wednesday:

Thursday:

Friday:

Saturday:

Sunday:

TIME TRACKER (optional)	HEALTHY FOOD 9-SQUARE	WRITER & ARTIST'S CORNER
Color in a section for every 10 minutes of exercise you have completed each day. Goal: 1 hour of daily exercise.	Make a smile face or place a sticker for every healthy food, found in this book, that you've eaten this week.	Make a sketch or write down thoughts about your exercise or healthy eating this week. Possible topics include: goals, nature, and food.

M
T
W
H
F
S
S

CYCLE ⊙ ⊙

Reason to Cycle "Power" Cycling makes your legs stonger.

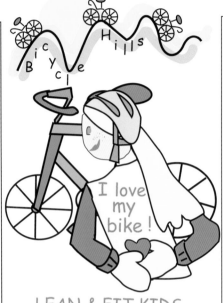

FUN FEET
Cycle

Pedal hard going uphill.

Let your bike coast downhill.

Spin your pedals fast on a flat.

Ride your bike often.

PACK-A-SNACK
Banana-split

whole banana
6 fresh strawberries
2 Tbsp walnuts
2 Tbsp vanilla ice cream
1 tsp chocolate chips

Put the whole banana into a dish. Top with the other ingredients. Add a sliced peach for a special treat.

LEAN & FIT KIDS
eat bananas before they ride!

GOOD STUFF
Bananas

-Vitamins B_6 and C to keep infection away

-Potassium to prevent cramps

-Great before- and after-exercise snack

-Yummy with healthy peanut butter

Monday's date _____

PHYSICAL ACTIVITY LOG

Record your physical activity for each day of the week. Older kids, record all of your physical activity. (Ex: Ran a mile with Dad. Rode my bike a block to Drew's house.) Younger kids, write at least one word to indicate your physical activity. (Ex: Soccer)

Monday:

Tuesday:

Wednesday:

Thursday:

Friday:

Saturday:

Sunday:

TIME TRACKER (optional)	HEALTHY FOOD 9-SQUARE	WRITER & ARTIST'S CORNER
Color in a section for every 10 minutes of exercise you have completed each day. Goal: 1 hour of daily exercise.	Make a smile face or place a sticker for every healthy food, found in this book, that you've eaten this week.	Make a sketch or write down thoughts about your exercise or healthy eating this week. Possible topics include: goals, nature, and food.

M
T
W
H
F
S
S

PLAY BASEBALL

Reason to Play Baseball "Pretend" It's fun to imagine you're a baseball star with big dreams.

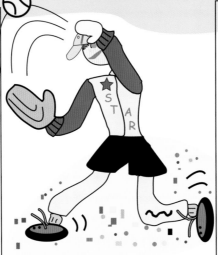

FUN FEET
Baseball
Skip and throw.

Swing, then hit.

Sprint and slide.

Do a victory jog around the bases.

LEAN & FIT KIDS
eat natural food.

PACK-A-SNACK
Berries
Strawberries

Blackberries

Raspberries

Blueberries

Cranberries

Use a rainbow of berries in a smoothie.

GOOD STUFF
Berries
-Lots of vitamin C

-Low calories

-Buy organic or grow your own.

-Don't use pesticides.

Monday's date _____

PHYSICAL ACTIVITY LOG

Record your physical activity for each day of the week. Older kids, record all of your physical activity. (Ex: Ran a mile with Dad. Rode my bike a block to Drew's house.) Younger kids, write at least one word to indicate your physical activity. (Ex: Soccer)

Monday:

Tuesday:

Wednesday:

Thursday:

Friday:

Saturday:

Sunday:

TIME TRACKER (optional)
Color in a section for every 10 minutes of exercise you have completed each day. Goal: 1 hour of daily exercise.

HEALTHY FOOD 9-SQUARE
Make a smile face or place a sticker for every healthy food, found in this book, that you've eaten this week.

WRITER & ARTIST'S CORNER
Make a sketch or write down thoughts about your exercise or healthy eating this week. Possible topics include: goals, nature, and food.

M
T
W
H
F
S
S

CRUNCH

Reason to Crunch "Strength" You will have strong abs.

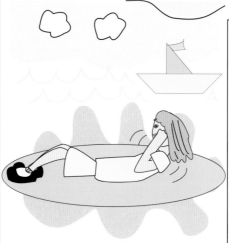

FUN FEET
Crunch
Feet flat

Knees bent

Arms as
shown or
crossed
over chest

Tighten your
stomach.

Lift your
upper body.

PACK-A-SNACK
Avocados
Sliced thin
on sandwiches

In guacamole
dip with
low-fat chips

Eat plain with
a little salt.

LEAN & FIT KIDS
do crunches at the
beach.

GOOD STUFF
Avocados
-Full of healthy fat

-Help keep cholesterol low

-Potassium and lots of vitamins

-Eat often, but keep portions small.

Monday's date _____

PHYSICAL ACTIVITY LOG

Record your physical activity for each day of the week. Older kids, record all of your physical activity. (Ex: Ran a mile with Dad. Rode my bike a block to Drew's house.) Younger kids, write at least one word to indicate your physical activity. (Ex: Soccer)

Monday:

Tuesday:

Wednesday:

Thursday:

Friday:

Saturday:

Sunday:

TIME TRACKER (optional)	HEALTHY FOOD 9-SQUARE	WRITER & ARTIST'S CORNER
Color in a section for every 10 minutes of exercise you have completed each day. Goal: 1 hour of daily exercise.	Make a smile face or place a sticker for every healthy food, found in this book, that you've eaten this week.	Make a sketch or write down thoughts about your exercise or healthy eating this week. Possible topics include: goals, nature, and food.

M
T
W
H
F
S
S

PLAY BASKETBALL

Reason to Play Basketball "Just for Fun" Sometimes it's more fun to play at home without pressure from a team.

FUN FEET
Basketball
Run and dribble.

Pivot and pass.

Do a jump shot.

"Swish" ... nothing but net.

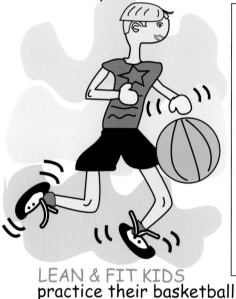

LEAN & FIT KIDS practice their basketball skills after school.

PACK-A-SNACK
Nuts
Peanuts

Almonds

Cashew nuts

Macadamia nuts

Brazil nuts

Walnuts

GOOD STUFF
Nuts
-Healthy fat and fiber

-No cholesterol

-Salty nuts with water are good if you are sweating a lot. Add a sports drink if you're at it for hours.

Monday's date _____

PHYSICAL ACTIVITY LOG

Record your physical activity for each day of the week. Older kids, record all of your physical activity. (Ex: Ran a mile with Dad. Rode my bike a block to Drew's house.) Younger kids, write at least one word to indicate your physical activity. (Ex: Soccer)

Monday:

Tuesday:

Wednesday:

Thursday:

Friday:

Saturday:

Sunday:

TIME TRACKER (optional)

Color in a section for every 10 minutes of exercise you have completed each day. Goal: 1 hour of daily exercise.

M
T
W
H
F
S
S

HEALTHY FOOD 9-SQUARE

Make a smile face or place a sticker for every healthy food, found in this book, that you've eaten this week.

WRITER & ARTIST'S CORNER

Make a sketch or write down thoughts about your exercise or healthy eating this week. Possible topics include: goals, nature, and food.

DANCE

Reason to Dance "Expression" Dance is a way to show your emotions through movement.

FUN FEET
Ballet
Learn the "Pas de chat"-step of the cat & "Pas de cheval"-step of the horse.

Stretch with an arabesque.

Spin with a pirouette.

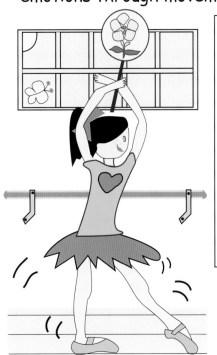

PACK-A-SNACK
Grapes
Green

Red

Purple

Seedless or seeded

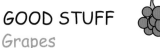

GOOD STUFF
Grapes
-Good for your heart

-Vitamin C

-Low in calories

-Fun to eat

Monday's date _____

PHYSICAL ACTIVITY LOG

Record your physical activity for each day of the week. Older kids, record all of your physical activity. (Ex: Ran a mile with Dad. Rode my bike a block to Drew's house.) Younger kids, write at least one word to indicate your physical activity. (Ex: Soccer)

Monday:	
Tuesday:	
Wednesday:	
Thursday:	
Friday:	
Saturday:	
Sunday:	

TIME TRACKER (optional)
Color in a section for every 10 minutes of exercise you have completed each day. Goal: 1 hour of daily exercise.

HEALTHY FOOD 9-SQUARE
Make a smile face or place a sticker for every healthy food, found in this book, that you've eaten this week.

WRITER & ARTIST'S CORNER
Make a sketch or write down thoughts about your exercise or healthy eating this week. Possible topics include: goals, nature, and food.

M
T
W
H
F
S
S

RUN TO WRITE

Reason to Run to Write "Love" You'll learn to love to write, just as you love to run.

FUN FEET
Run to Write
Run, then write about your run in a journal.

Write an adventure story about running in a maze.

Create poetry to the rhythm of your run.

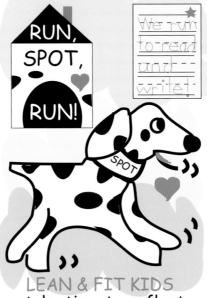

RUN, SPOT, RUN!

We run to read and write!

LEAN & FIT KIDS take time to reflect on their fitness.

PACK-A-SNACK
Salsa

6 chopped cherry tomatoes
1/4 c chopped cucumbers
1/4 c chopped bell peppers
1 tsp lime juice
dash of garlic salt
1 tsp chopped and stemmed jalapeno pepper

Mix ingredients together. Keep refrigerated. Eat plain, with chips, or with bean burritos.

GOOD STUFF
Tomatoes

-Almost fat free

-Low in calories

-Lots of vitamin C

-May help to prevent cancer

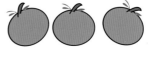

Monday's date _____

PHYSICAL ACTIVITY LOG

Record your physical activity for each day of the week. Older kids, record all of your physical activity. (Ex: Ran a mile with Dad. Rode my bike a block to Drew's house.) Younger kids, write at least one word to indicate your physical activity. (Ex: Soccer)

Monday:

Tuesday:

Wednesday:

Thursday:

Friday:

Saturday:

Sunday:

TIME TRACKER
(optional)
Color in a section for every 10 minutes of exercise you have completed each day. Goal: 1 hour of daily exercise.

M
T
W
H
F
S
S

HEALTHY FOOD
9-SQUARE
Make a smile face or place a sticker for every healthy food, found in this book, that you've eaten this week.

WRITER & ARTIST'S
CORNER
Make a sketch or write down thoughts about your exercise or healthy eating this week. Possible topics include: goals, nature, and food.

RUN

Reason to Run "Nature" Delight your senses with the wonders of nature. Start with the sense of sight.

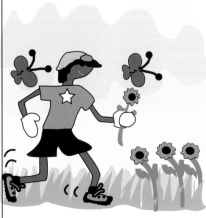

FUN FEET
Run

Smell the first signs of spring.

Feel your footsteps in the summer.

Hear the leaves crunch in the fall.

Taste falling snow in the winter.

LEAN & FIT KIDS
stay active in all of the seasons: summer, fall, winter, and spring.

PACK-A-SNACK
Whole-wheat Muffins

Change any muffin recipe by using some whole-wheat flour instead of enriched flour.

Cookies

Do the same with any cookie recipe.

GOOD STUFF
Whole-wheat

-Has calcium, fiber, and protein

-May help prevent cancer

-Calcium helps build strong bones.

-Eat whole-wheat pancakes.

Monday's date _____

PHYSICAL ACTIVITY LOG

Record your physical activity for each day of the week. Older kids, record all of your physical activity. (Ex: Ran a mile with Dad. Rode my bike a block to Drew's house.) Younger kids, write at least one word to indicate your physical activity. (Ex: Soccer)

Monday:

Tuesday:

Wednesday:

Thursday:

Friday:

Saturday:

Sunday:

TIME TRACKER (optional)
Color in a section for every 10 minutes of exercise you have completed each day. Goal: 1 hour of daily exercise.

HEALTHY FOOD 9-SQUARE
Make a smile face or place a sticker for every healthy food, found in this book, that you've eaten this week.

WRITER & ARTIST'S CORNER
Make a sketch or write down thoughts about your exercise or healthy eating this week. Possible topics include: goals, nature, and food.

M
T
W
H
F
S
S

SWIM

Reason to Swim "Heartbeat" Swimming is good for your heart.

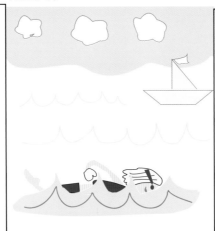

FUN FEET
Kick

Do the crawl and kick.

Hold a flutter board and kick.

Hold on to the side of the pool and kick.

LEAN & FIT KIDS
choose swimming over sunbathing.

PACK-A-SNACK
Low-fat Yogurt

Frozen or non-frozen

Blueberry

Strawberry

Lime

Cherry

Lemon

GOOD STUFF
Yogurt

-Vitamin B_{12} for healthy nerves and blood

-Calcium for strong teeth and bones

-Use yogurt in fruit smoothies for a nutritiously sweet treat.

Monday's date _____

PHYSICAL ACTIVITY LOG

Record your physical activity for each day of the week. Older kids, record all of your physical activity. (Ex: Ran a mile with Dad. Rode my bike a block to Drew's house.) Younger kids, write at least one word to indicate your physical activity. (Ex: Soccer)

Monday:

Tuesday:

Wednesday:

Thursday:

Friday:

Saturday:

Sunday:

TIME TRACKER (optional)	HEALTHY FOOD 9-SQUARE	WRITER & ARTIST'S CORNER
Color in a section for every 10 minutes of exercise you have completed each day. Goal: 1 hour of daily exercise.	Make a smile face or place a sticker for every healthy food, found in this book, that you've eaten this week.	Make a sketch or write down thoughts about your exercise or healthy eating this week. Possible topics include: goals, nature, and food.

M
T
W
H
F
S
S

WALK

Reason to Walk "Lifelong Exercise" Walking is a healthy activity for people of all ages.

FUN FEET
Walk

Walk with your family.

Walk to the post office.

Walk to the store.

Walk to the restaurant.

Walk everywhere.

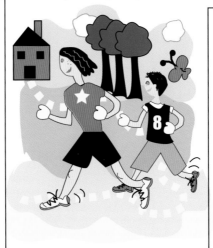

LEAN & FIT KIDS
walk whenever they can.

PACK-A-SNACK
Bell Peppers

Red peppers

Green peppers

Yellow peppers

Orange peppers

Purple peppers

GOOD STUFF
Bell Peppers
-Lots of vitamins C and A

-Low in calories

-The red peppers have the most vitamins.

-Eat plain, in pasta sauce, and in salads.

Monday's date _____

PHYSICAL ACTIVITY LOG

Record your physical activity for each day of the week. Older kids, record all of your physical activity. (Ex: Ran a mile with Dad. Rode my bike a block to Drew's house.) Younger kids, write at least one word to indicate your physical activity. (Ex: Soccer)

Monday:

Tuesday:

Wednesday:

Thursday:

Friday:

Saturday:

Sunday:

TIME TRACKER
(optional)
Color in a section for every 10 minutes of exercise you have completed each day. Goal: 1 hour of daily exercise.

HEALTHY FOOD
9-SQUARE
Make a smile face or place a sticker for every healthy food, found in this book, that you've eaten this week.

WRITER & ARTIST'S
CORNER
Make a sketch or write down thoughts about your exercise or healthy eating this week. Possible topics include: goals, nature, and food.

PLAY BALL

Reason to Play Ball "Full-body Exercise" You'll work your arms, legs, torso, and feet.

FUN FEET
Play Ball

Kick a soccer ball.

Punt a football.

Kick a kickball.

Run with a football.

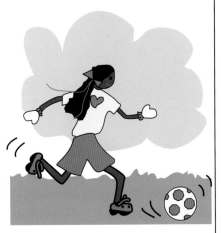

LEAN & FIT KIDS eat lean meat to restore muscle.

PACK-A-SNACK
Half-sandwich

Lean turkey

Whole-wheat bread

Lettuce

Tomatoes

Peppers

Sprouts

Mustard

GOOD STUFF
Lean Meat

-Protein to build muscle

-B vitamins for healthy skin and blood

-Ask for lean meat at the deli. The closer to 100% fat free, the leaner the meat is.

PHYSICAL ACTIVITY LOG

Record your physical activity for each day of the week. Older kids, record all of your physical activity. (Ex: Ran a mile with Dad. Rode my bike a block to Drew's house.) Younger kids, write at least one word to indicate your physical activity. (Ex: Soccer)

Monday:

Tuesday:

Wednesday:

Thursday:

Friday:

Saturday:

Sunday:

TIME TRACKER (optional)
Color in a section for every 10 minutes of exercise you have completed each day. Goal: 1 hour of daily exercise.

HEALTHY FOOD 9-SQUARE
Make a smile face or place a sticker for every healthy food, found in this book, that you've eaten this week.

WRITER & ARTIST'S CORNER
Make a sketch or write down thoughts about your exercise or healthy eating this week. Possible topics include: goals, nature, and food.

M
T
W
T
F
S
S

SNOWSHOE

Reason to Snowshoe "Beauty" You might see a deer.

FUN FEET
Snowshoe
Walk in the deep snow.

Run across an open field.

Climb up a steep hill.

Follow a rabbit's trail.

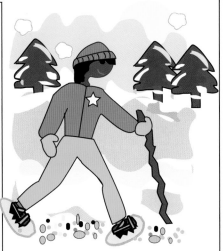

LEAN & FIT KIDS
love winter sports.

PACK-A-SNACK
Beans
Pinto beans

Black beans

Navy beans

Soybeans

Split peas

Lima beans

Chick-peas

GOOD STUFF
Beans
-Lots of fiber and B vitamins

-Filling

-Low in fat

-May help you lower cholesterol

Monday's date _____

PHYSICAL ACTIVITY LOG

Record your physical activity for each day of the week. Older kids, record all of your physical activity. (Ex: Ran a mile with Dad. Rode my bike a block to Drew's house.) Younger kids, write at least one word to indicate your physical activity. (Ex: Soccer)

Monday:

Tuesday:

Wednesday:

Thursday:

Friday:

Saturday:

Sunday:

TIME TRACKER (optional)	HEALTHY FOOD 9-SQUARE	WRITER & ARTIST'S CORNER
Color in a section for every 10 minutes of exercise you have completed each day. Goal: 1 hour of daily exercise.	Make a smile face or place a sticker for every healthy food, found in this book, that you've eaten this week.	Make a sketch or write down thoughts about your exercise or healthy eating this week. Possible topics include: goals, nature, and food.

M
T
W
T
F
S
S

YOGA

Reason to Practice Yoga "Energy" You will feel refreshed.

FUN FEET
Yoga

Be confident through standing postures.

Be flexible through seated postures.

Strengthen your body with all postures.

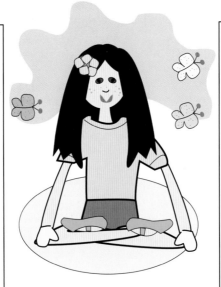

LEAN & FIT KIDS
take care of their bodies and minds.

PACK-A-SNACK
Rice

Brown rice with vegetables

Wild rice with chicken

White rice balls wrapped with seaweed

Rice pudding made with low-fat milk

GOOD STUFF
Rice

-High in carbohydrates

-Low in fat and no cholesterol

-Brown rice and wild rice are more nutritious than white rice.

Monday's date _____

PHYSICAL ACTIVITY LOG

Record your physical activity for each day of the week. Older kids, record all of your physical activity. (Ex: Ran a mile with Dad. Rode my bike a block to Drew's house.) Younger kids, write at least one word to indicate your physical activity. (Ex: Soccer)

Monday:

Tuesday:

Wednesday:

Thursday:

Friday:

Saturday:

Sunday:

TIME TRACKER (optional)

Color in a section for every 10 minutes of exercise you have completed each day. Goal: 1 hour of daily exercise.

HEALTHY FOOD 9-SQUARE

Make a smile face or place a sticker for every healthy food, found in this book, that you've eaten this week.

WRITER & ARTIST'S CORNER

Make a sketch or write down thoughts about your exercise or healthy eating this week. Possible topics include: goals, nature, and food.

M
T
W
H
F
S
S

RUN

Reason to Run "Focus" Running helps use up energy so that you can settle down and do your homework.

FUN FEET
Veggie Tag
Run in the "paddock".

When you're tagged, go to the "garden".

Call out or write the name of a vegetable and then you're it!

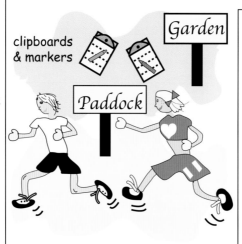

clipboards & markers

Garden

Paddock

LEAN & FIT KIDS
eat green veggies.

PACK-A-SNACK
Broccoli Pizza

1/2 English muffin
2 Tbsp tomato sauce
1 Tbsp low-fat cheese
1 Tbsp steamed broccoli

Spread tomato sauce on English muffin. Top with cheese and broccoli. Microwave until warm.

GOOD STUFF
Broccoli
-Vitamin C

-Vitamin A

-May help protect you from cancer

-Eat fresh broccoli with a low-fat dip.

Monday's date _____

PHYSICAL ACTIVITY LOG

Record your physical activity for each day of the week. Older kids, record all of your physical activity. (Ex: Ran a mile with Dad. Rode my bike a block to Drew's house.) Younger kids, write at least one word to indicate your physical activity. (Ex: Soccer)

Monday:

Tuesday:

Wednesday:

Thursday:

Friday:

Saturday:

Sunday:

TIME TRACKER (optional)	HEALTHY FOOD 9-SQUARE	WRITER & ARTIST'S CORNER
Color in a section for every 10 minutes of exercise you have completed each day. Goal: 1 hour of daily exercise.	Make a smile face or place a sticker for every healthy food, found in this book, that you've eaten this week.	Make a sketch or write down thoughts about your exercise or healthy eating this week. Possible topics include: goals, nature, and food.

M
T
W
H
F
S
S

JUMP ROPE

Reason to Jump Rope "Bones" Jumping when you are young, builds strong bones.

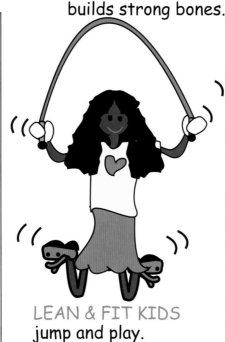

FUN FEET
Jump Rope
Count by 5's.

Say a rhyme.

Jump ten times.

Jump to a beat.

A, B, C, D, E, F, G...

"Skip" rope.

LEAN & FIT KIDS
jump and play.

PACK-A-SNACK
Peanut Butter
Apple

1 cored apple
1 Tbsp peanut butter
cinnamon, nutmeg, or alspice
1 Tbsp vanilla yogurt

Fill the apple with peanut butter. Sprinkle with a spice. Wrap in plastic wrap. Microwave until soft (about 1-2 minutes). Top with yogurt.

GOOD STUFF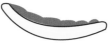
Peanut Butter

-B vitamins, protein, and fat (Kids need a higher percentage of fat than adults, but the fat should be healthy fat.)

-Choose peanut butter which has oil separated on top. Just stir before you use. Look for "No trans fatty acids" on the label.

-Make sandwiches with peanut butter and sliced bananas instead of jelly.

Monday's date _____

PHYSICAL ACTIVITY LOG

Record your physical activity for each day of the week. Older kids, record all of your physical activity. (Ex: Ran a mile with Dad. Rode my bike a block to Drew's house.) Younger kids, write at least one word to indicate your physical activity. (Ex: Soccer)

Monday:

Tuesday:

Wednesday:

Thursday:

Friday:

Saturday:

Sunday:

TIME TRACKER (optional)

Color in a section for every 10 minutes of exercise you have completed each day. Goal: 1 hour of daily exercise.

HEALTHY FOOD 9-SQUARE

Make a smile face or place a sticker for every healthy food, found in this book, that you've eaten this week.

WRITER & ARTIST'S CORNER

Make a sketch or write down thoughts about your exercise or healthy eating this week. Possible topics include: goals, nature, and food.

M
T
W
T
F
S
S

RUN

Reason to Run   "Marathon Dream" If your heart is full of desire, and you stick with your running, you can finish a marathon when you grow up.

FUN FEET
Marathon
Enter fun runs as often as you can.

While you're running, pretend you're in a marathon.

Go to road races and cheer on the runners.

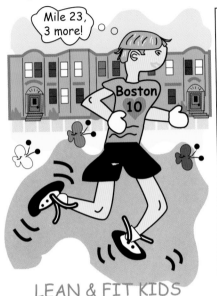

Mile 23, 3 more!

Boston 10

LEAN & FIT KIDS
have short- and long-term goals.

PACK-A-SNACK
Pasta Salad

1/2 c cooled pasta
1 tsp olive oil
1/4 c chopped celery
1/4 c chopped red bell pepper
dash of salt, dill, and pepper

Mix together. Refrigerate.

This recipe makes a good day-before-the-race snack.

GOOD STUFF
Pasta
-Low fat, low or no cholesterol

-Thiamine and iron for energy

-Spaghetti, Linguine (little tongues), Capellini (angel hair), Conghiglie (shells), Penne (quills), Stelline (little stars), and Farfalle (bow ties or butterflies)

Monday's date _____

PHYSICAL ACTIVITY LOG

Record your physical activity for each day of the week. Older kids, record all of your physical activity. (Ex: Ran a mile with Dad. Rode my bike a block to Drew's house.) Younger kids, write at least one word to indicate your physical activity. (Ex: Soccer)

Monday:

Tuesday:

Wednesday:

Thursday:

Friday:

Saturday:

Sunday:

TIME TRACKER
(optional)
Color in a section for every 10 minutes of exercise you have completed each day. Goal: 1 hour of daily exercise.

HEALTHY FOOD 9-SQUARE
Make a smile face or place a sticker for every healthy food, found in this book, that you've eaten this week.

WRITER & ARTIST'S CORNER
Make a sketch or write down thoughts about your exercise or healthy eating this week. Possible topics include: goals, nature, and food.

M
T
W
T
F
S
S

ENTER A CHARITABLE EVENT

Reason to Fund Raise "Save Lives" The money you raise may help find a cure for disease.

FUN FEET
Charity
Cycle with a kids' event for Dana Farber.

Run a fun run at a Race for the Cure.

Do Jump Rope for Heart.

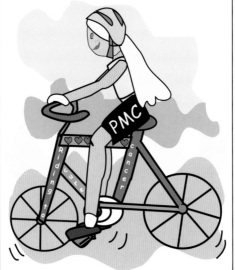

LEAN & FIT KIDS train for events.

PACK-A-SNACK
Baked Potato
Bake in the microwave or oven.

Top with low-fat cottage cheese, veggies, and spices.

Add a little salt and pepper.

GOOD STUFF
Baked Potato
-Fiber

-Complex carbohydrates for lots of continued energy

-Lots of potassium

Monday's date _____

PHYSICAL ACTIVITY LOG

Record your physical activity for each day of the week. Older kids, record all of your physical activity. (Ex: Ran a mile with Dad. Rode my bike a block to Drew's house.) Younger kids, write at least one word to indicate your physical activity. (Ex: Soccer)

Monday:

Tuesday:

Wednesday:

Thursday:

Friday:

Saturday:

Sunday:

TIME TRACKER (optional)

Color in a section for every 10 minutes of exercise you have completed each day. Goal: 1 hour of daily exercise.

HEALTHY FOOD 9-SQUARE

Make a smile face or place a sticker for every healthy food, found in this book, that you've eaten this week.

WRITER & ARTIST'S CORNER

Make a sketch or write down thoughts about your exercise or healthy eating this week. Possible topics include: goals, nature, and food.

M
T
W
H
F
S
S

PLAY HOPSCOTCH

Reason to Play Hopscotch "Agility" Hopscotch uses quick, light hops and jumps.

FUN FEET
Hopscotch

Throw a marker.

Hop over the marker.

Hop with one foot.

Jump with two.

Turn around.

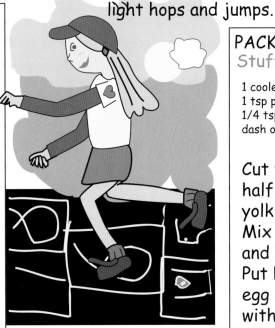

LEAN & FIT KIDS
can play all day.

PACK-A-SNACK
Stuffed Eggs

1 cooled hard boiled egg
1 tsp plain low-fat yogurt
1/4 tsp mustard
dash of dill and paprika

Cut the egg in half. Remove the yolk and mash. Mix with yogurt and mustard. Put back into egg whites. Top with dill and paprika. Keep refrigerated.

GOOD STUFF
Eggs
-Protein

-B vitamins and vitamin A

-Caution: High in cholesterol
This is a concern for kids who are cholesterol sensitive.

Monday's date _____

Record your physical activity for each day of the week. Older kids, record all of your physical activity. (Ex: Ran a mile with Dad. Rode my bike a block to Drew's house.) Younger kids, write at least one word to indicate your physical activity. (Ex: Soccer)

Monday:

Tuesday:

Wednesday:

Thursday:

Friday:

Saturday:

Sunday:

TIME TRACKER (optional)

Color in a section for every 10 minutes of exercise you have completed each day. Goal: 1 hour of daily exercise.

HEALTHY FOOD 9-SQUARE

Make a smile face or place a sticker for every healthy food, found in this book, that you've eaten this week.

WRITER & ARTIST'S CORNER

Make a sketch or write down thoughts about your exercise or healthy eating this week. Possible topics include: goals, nature, and food.

CROSS-COUNTRY SKI

Reason to Ski "Lungs" Cross-country skiing is a great aerobic workout. It will help your lungs do their job.

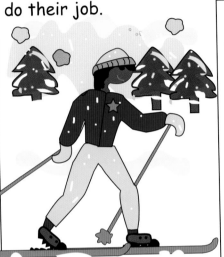

FUN FEET
Cross-Country Ski

Slide your right foot forward.

Slide your left foot forward.

Climb uphill.

Glide down-hill.

LEAN & FIT KIDS love the exhilaration of exercising in cold weather.

PACK-A-SNACK
Hot Chocolate

1 tsp unsweetened cocoa
1 tsp sugar
1 c low-fat milk

Mix cocoa, sugar, and 2 Tbsp milk in a cup. Add the rest of the milk. Microwave 1 1/2 minutes. Serve with 5 animal crackers and 2 or 3 banana wheels.

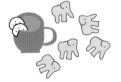

GOOD STUFF
Low-fat Milk

-Low in fat

-Vitamins C, A, B_2, and B_{12}

-Calcium for strong bones

-Protein

Monday's date _____

PHYSICAL ACTIVITY LOG

Record your physical activity for each day of the week. Older kids, record all of your physical activity. (Ex: Ran a mile with Dad. Rode my bike a block to Drew's house.) Younger kids, write at least one word to indicate your physical activity. (Ex: Soccer)

Monday:

Tuesday:

Wednesday:

Thursday:

Friday:

Saturday:

Sunday:

TIME TRACKER (optional)	HEALTHY FOOD 9-SQUARE	WRITER & ARTIST'S CORNER
Color in a section for every 10 minutes of exercise you have completed each day. Goal: 1 hour of daily exercise.	Make a smile face or place a sticker for every healthy food, found in this book, that you've eaten this week.	Make a sketch or write down thoughts about your exercise or healthy eating this week. Possible topics include: goals, nature, and food.

ICE SKATE

Reason to Ice Skate "Grace" Ice skating is a combination of exercise and graceful moves.

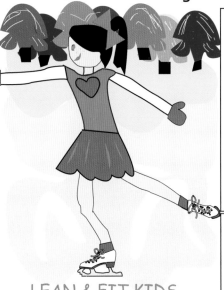

FUN FEET
Ice Skate
Push off to start.

Glide on both skates.

Stroke the ice.

Wiggle to skate backward.

LEAN & FIT KIDS
find art in athletics.

PACK-A-SNACK
Chicken Vege-table Soup

2 c low-fat chicken broth
1/4 c cooked chicken chunks
1/4 c cooked celery
1/4 c cooked carrots
1/4 c cooked corn
1/4 c cooked tomatoes
1/4 c cooked peas
1/4 c cooked spinach

Heat in pot till warm. Pack in thermos. Eat with saltine crackers.

GOOD STUFF
Chicken Vegetable Soup

-Some protein

-Rich in vitamins A, C, and B

-It's fun to add your favorite vegetables.

Monday's date _____

PHYSICAL ACTIVITY LOG

Record your physical activity for each day of the week. Older kids, record all of your physical activity. (Ex: Ran a mile with Dad. Rode my bike a block to Drew's house.) Younger kids, write at least one word to indicate your physical activity. (Ex: Soccer)

Monday:

Tuesday:

Wednesday:

Thursday:

Friday:

Saturday:

Sunday:

TIME TRACKER (optional)

Color in a section for every 10 minutes of exercise you have completed each day. Goal: 1 hour of daily exercise.

HEALTHY FOOD 9-SQUARE

Make a smile face or place a sticker for every healthy food, found in this book, that you've eaten this week.

WRITER & ARTIST'S CORNER

Make a sketch or write down thoughts about your exercise or healthy eating this week. Possible topics include: goals, nature, and food.

M
T
W
H
F
S
S

PLAY TENNIS

Reason to Play Tennis

"Concentration" You'll learn to focus and react quickly on the court.

FUN FEET
Tennis

Hit the ball against a wall.

Play on a court.

Practice your foot-work.

Do crossovers and sidesteps.

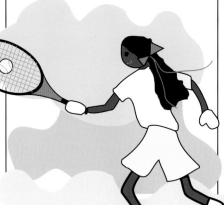

LEAN & FIT KIDS
like sports which keep them moving.

PACK-A-SNACK
Watermelon

Just a plain slice

In fruit salad

Mixed into vanilla yogurt

Eat as a snack, or with break-fast, lunch, or dinner.

GOOD STUFF
Watermelon
-Low in calories

-Lots of vitamin C

-Some vitamin A

-No cholesterol

Monday's date _____

PHYSICAL ACTIVITY LOG

Record your physical activity for each day of the week. Older kids, record all of your physical activity. (Ex: Ran a mile with Dad. Rode my bike a block to Drew's house.) Younger kids, write at least one word to indicate your physical activity. (Ex: Soccer)

Monday:

Tuesday:

Wednesday:

Thursday:

Friday:

Saturday:

Sunday:

TIME TRACKER (optional)	HEALTHY FOOD 9-SQUARE	WRITER & ARTIST'S CORNER
Color in a section for every 10 minutes of exercise you have completed each day. Goal: 1 hour of daily exercise.	Make a smile face or place a sticker for every healthy food, found in this book, that you've eaten this week.	Make a sketch or write down thoughts about your exercise or healthy eating this week. Possible topics include: goals, nature, and food.

M
T
W
H
F
S
S

PICK PUMPKINS

Reason to Pick Pumpkins "Halloween" You can find a perfect pumpkin for your jack-o'-lantern.

FUN FEET
Pick Pumpkins
Walk to the pumpkin patch.

Walk up and down the rows to see all of the pumpkins.

Pick out your favorite pumpkin.

If you can, carry it home.

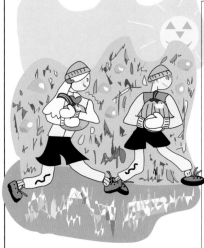

LEAN & FIT KIDS love to walk around the pumpkin patch.

PACK-A-SNACK
Pumpkin Pie
Crust
1 c whole-wheat pastry flour
4 Tbsp canola oil
3 Tbsp ice water

Mix and press into pie pan.

Filling
1 can pumpkin
1 c skim milk
3 eggs
6 Tbsp brown sugar
1/2 tsp cinnamon and nutmeg
1/4 tsp salt

Mix, pour into pan bake at 350° for 1 hr. or until firm.

GOOD STUFF
Pumpkin
-Vitamin A

- Iron

-Vitamin C

-Low in fat

Monday's date _____

PHYSICAL ACTIVITY LOG

Record your physical activity for each day of the week. Older kids, record all of your physical activity. (Ex: Ran a mile with Dad. Rode my bike a block to Drew's house.) Younger kids, write at least one word to indicate your physical activity. (Ex: Soccer)

Monday:

Tuesday:

Wednesday:

Thursday:

Friday:

Saturday:

Sunday:

TIME TRACKER (optional)	HEALTHY FOOD 9-SQUARE	WRITER & ARTIST'S CORNER
Color in a section for every 10 minutes of exercise you have completed each day. Goal: 1 hour of daily exercise.	Make a smile face or place a sticker for every healthy food, found in this book, that you've eaten this week.	Make a sketch or write down thoughts about your exercise or healthy eating this week. Possible topics include: goals, nature, and food.

M
T
W
H
F
S
S

PUSH-UPS

Reason to Do Push-ups "Just your Body" You don't need any special equipment. You can do push-ups anywhere.

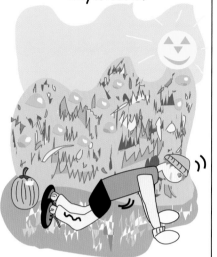

FUN FEET
Push-ups
Start with push-ups on your knees.

Later, do them on your toes.

Use your arms to raise and lower your body.

LEAN & FIT KIDS
use their own body weight as resistance.

PACK-A-SNACK
Pumpkin Seeds

washed pumpkin seeds from 1 pumpkin
salt to taste
seasoning-optional
(cinnamon, red pepper, curry, dill, guacamole spice, etc.)

Salt and season pumpkin seeds. Put on a cookie sheet. Bake at 250° until brown about 15-30 minutes.

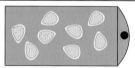

GOOD STUFF
Pumpkin Seeds
-Iron, magnesium, and zinc

-No cholesterol

-High in fat, but "healthy" fat so may help with cholesterol

Monday's date _____

PHYSICAL ACTIVITY LOG

Record your physical activity for each day of the week. Older kids, record all of your physical activity. (Ex: Ran a mile with Dad. Rode my bike a block to Drew's house.) Younger kids, write at least one word to indicate your physical activity. (Ex: Soccer)

Monday:

Tuesday:

Wednesday:

Thursday:

Friday:

Saturday:

Sunday:

TIME TRACKER (optional)
Color in a section for every 10 minutes of exercise you have completed each day. Goal: 1 hour of daily exercise.

HEALTHY FOOD 9-SQUARE
Make a smile face or place a sticker for every healthy food, found in this book, that you've eaten this week.

WRITER & ARTIST'S CORNER
Make a sketch or write down thoughts about your exercise or healthy eating this week. Possible topics include: goals, nature, and food.

Kids   Dogs

TRAIN YOUR PET

Reason to Train your Pet "Obedience" If your dog is under control, you can exercise with it at a park.

FUN FEET
Training

Teach your dog to walk on a leash.

Teach your dog to fetch.

Teach your dog to sit and stay.

Teach your dog to run by your side.

PACK-A-SNACK
RyKrisp
(for kids only)
Eat plain.

Eat with low-fat cottage cheese.

Eat with healthy peanut butter.

Dog Treats
(for dogs only)
Use to reward dogs during training.

LEAN & FIT KIDS
exercise by themselves, AND with their friends, families, and pets.

GOOD STUFF
RyKrisp

-Low in fat and no cholesterol

-Fiber

-Magnesium for good blood pressure

-Zinc for healthy skin

Monday's date _____

PHYSICAL ACTIVITY LOG

Record your physical activity for each day of the week. Older kids, record all of your physical activity. (Ex: Ran a mile with Dad. Rode my bike a block to Drew's house.) Younger kids, write at least one word to indicate your physical activity. (Ex: Soccer)

Monday:
Tuesday:
Wednesday:
Thursday:
Friday:
Saturday:
Sunday:

TIME TRACKER (optional)

Color in a section for every 10 minutes of exercise you have completed each day. Goal: 1 hour of daily exercise.

HEALTHY FOOD 9-SQUARE

Make a smile face or place a sticker for every healthy food, found in this book, that you've eaten this week.

WRITER & ARTIST'S CORNER

Make a sketch or write down thoughts about your exercise or healthy eating this week. Possible topics include: goals, nature, and food.

TEAM
Reason to Join a Team "Camaraderie" A team can be a circle of true friendship.

FUN FEET
Team

You can enter the Junior Olympics.

You can learn new skills.

You can help your team-mates.

You can work out often.

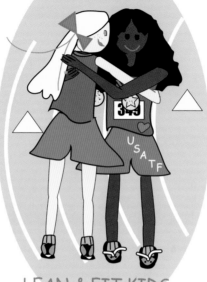

LEAN & FIT KIDS compete with the goal of doing their best.

PACK-A-SNACK
Quesadilla

1 healthy tortilla wrap
1/2 c sliced mushrooms
1/4 c chopped onions.
1/4 c red bell pepper
4 chopped black olives
1 Tbsp shredded carrots
1 Tbsp corn kernels
2 Tbsp grated low-fat
cheddar cheese
1/4 tsp chili powder
1 pinch curry powder
1 pinch salt

Saute veggies with spices. Place wrap on plate. Add veggies and cheese Fold. Microwave for 30 seconds.

GOOD STUFF
Mushrooms

-Low fat

-Fiber

-Niacin and iron for healthy blood

-Carbohydrates for slow release energy

Monday's date _____

PHYSICAL ACTIVITY LOG

Record your physical activity for each day of the week. Older kids, record all of your physical activity. (Ex: Ran a mile with Dad. Rode my bike a block to Drew's house.) Younger kids, write at least one word to indicate your physical activity. (Ex: Soccer)

Monday:

Tuesday:

Wednesday:

Thursday:

Friday:

Saturday:

Sunday:

TIME TRACKER (optional)	HEALTHY FOOD 9-SQUARE	WRITER & ARTIST'S CORNER
Color in a section for every 10 minutes of exercise you have completed each day. Goal: 1 hour of daily exercise.	Make a smile face or place a sticker for every healthy food, found in this book, that you've eaten this week.	Make a sketch or write down thoughts about your exercise or healthy eating this week. Possible topics include: goals, nature, and food.

M
T
W
T
F
S
S

CYCLE
Reason to Cycle "Go Places" Cycle to the peach festival with your big sister.

FUN FEET
Cycle
You can cycle on the trails to a frog pond.

You can cycle on the road to the park.

You can cycle on the path to a black-berry patch.

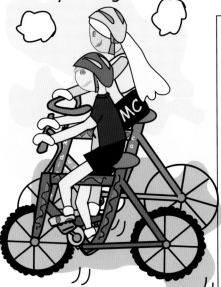

LEAN & FIT KIDS
cycle by the peach short-cake and choose a fresh peach instead.

PACK-A-SNACK
Peach
Eat a whole fresh peach.

Slice and sprinkle with cinnamon.

Eat with yogurt.

If you do bake a pie, go easy on (or eliminate) the sugar, and make a healthy pie crust.

GOOD STUFF
Peaches
-Low in fat

-Fiber

-Vitamin C

-Plant 2 peach trees and grow your own.

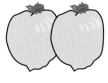

Monday's date _____

HYSICAL ACTIVITY LOG

ecord your physical activity for each day of the week. Older kids, record
ll of your physical activity. (Ex: Ran a mile with Dad. Rode my bike a block
o Drew's house.) Younger kids, write at least one word to indicate your
hysical activity. (Ex: Soccer)

Monday:

uesday:

Vednesday:

hursday:

riday:

aturday:

unday:

TIME TRACKER
(optional)
Color in a section for
every 10 minutes of
exercise you have
completed each day.
Goal: 1 hour of daily
exercise.

HEALTHY FOOD
9-SQUARE
Make a smile face or
place a sticker for
every healthy food,
found in this book,
that you've eaten this
week.

WRITER & ARTIST'S
CORNER
Make a sketch or write
down thoughts about
your exercise or healthy
eating this week. Possible
topics include: goals,
nature, and food.

TOUR

Reason to Tour "Sight-see" You can spend the day touring an outdoor museum and get your exercise at the same time.

FUN FEET
Tour

Walk , skip, or jog down the rustic paths.

Pump water, roll a hoop, and skip rocks into the river.

Enjoy the animals, landscape, and buildings.

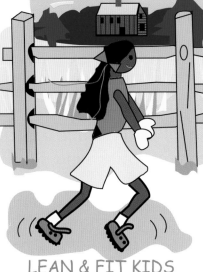

LEAN & FIT KIDS love family outings that involve physical activity and education.

PACK-A-SNACK
Sweet Potato Pancakes

1 c whole-wheat pastry flour
1 tsp brown sugar
1 tsp baking powder
1/2 tsp salt
3/4 c skim milk
1 egg
1 Tbsp canola oil
3 Tbsp cooked sweet potato
1 tsp cinnamon

Mix. Spray griddle with no-fat spray. Pour pancakes onto hot griddle. Flip when bubbles appear.

GOOD STUFF
Sweet Potatoes

-Vitamin A

-Vitamin C

-B vitamins

-Lots of fiber and carbohydrates

PHYSICAL ACTIVITY LOG

Record your physical activity for each day of the week. Older kids, record all of your physical activity. (Ex: Ran a mile with Dad. Rode my bike a block to Drew's house.) Younger kids, write at least one word to indicate your physical activity. (Ex: Soccer)

Monday:

Tuesday:

Wednesday:

Thursday:

Friday:

Saturday:

Sunday:

TIME TRACKER (optional)

Color in a section for every 10 minutes of exercise you have completed each day. Goal: 1 hour of daily exercise.

HEALTHY FOOD 9-SQUARE

Make a smile face or place a sticker for every healthy food, found in this book, that you've eaten this week.

WRITER & ARTIST'S CORNER

Make a sketch or write down thoughts about your exercise or healthy eating this week. Possible topics include: goals, nature, and food.

M
T
W
H
F
S
S

NATURE HUNT

Reason to Nature Hunt "Curiosity" You can run to capture a creature, closely observe it, then let it g...

FUN FEET
Nature Play
Run and net fireflies.

Sprint and chase wild turkeys.

Wade and catch cray-fish.

Hop and grab frogs.

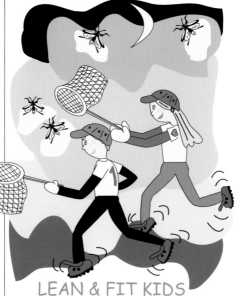

LEAN & FIT KIDS
take good care of our natural habitat.

PACK-A-SNACK
Lightning Bug Muffins
1 c yellow corn meal
1/2 c white flour
1/2 c buckwheat flour
2 tsp baking powder
1/2 tsp salt
2 Tbsp brown sugar
1 c plain Silk® soymilk
1 egg
a few dried dates
small can kernel corn
Preheat oven to 350°.
Mix dry ingredients.
Stir in soymilk and egg. Spray mini-muffin tins with Pam. Spoon in mix. Top with slices of dates (wings) and corn (lights). Bake 15 minutes or until done.

GOOD STUFF
Silk® Soymilk
- Low in fat, lactose free

- No cholesterol

- Vitamins A and D

- Calcium

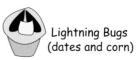

Lightning Bugs (dates and corn)

Red Butterflies (cherries and chocolate chips)

Swamp Milkweed Leaf Beetles (bananas and raisins)

This Fun Feet section was inspired by Rob, age 7, Birch Grove Primary School, Tolland, CT.

Monday's date _____

PHYSICAL ACTIVITY LOG

Record your physical activity for each day of the week. Older kids, record all of your physical activity. (Ex: Ran a mile with Dad. Rode my bike a block to Drew's house.) Younger kids, write at least one word to indicate your physical activity. (Ex: Soccer)

Monday:

Tuesday:

Wednesday:

Thursday:

Friday:

Saturday:

Sunday:

TIME TRACKER (optional)

Color in a section for every 10 minutes of exercise you have completed each day. Goal: 1 hour of daily exercise.

HEALTHY FOOD 9-SQUARE

Make a smile face or place a sticker for every healthy food, found in this book, that you've eaten this week.

WRITER & ARTIST'S CORNER

Make a sketch or write down thoughts about your exercise or healthy eating this week. Possible topics include: goals, nature, and food.

M
T
W
H
F
S
S

RUN A RELAY RACE

Reason to Relay "Rules" You can make up your own rules for a relay race. Just use your imagination.

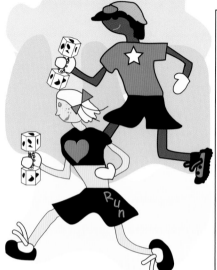

FUN FEET
Relay Races
Use dog-chew toys for safe batons.

At holiday time use festive "hot-oven mitts" instead of batons.

Add different types of locomotion.

LEAN & FIT KIDS
enjoy teamwork and show good sportsmanship.

PACK-A-SNACK
Salad Bar
Romaine lettuce
beets
shredded red cabbage
shredded carrots
cut up fresh broccoli
sliced cucumbers
endive
sliced bell peppers
radishes
fresh baby spinach
olive oil
vinegar
salt and pepper

Have each member of the relay team bring one or two of the ingredients. Then get in line and make your own salad.

GOOD STUFF
Romaine Lettuce
-Folate

-Vitamins C and A

-Fiber

-Low in fat and no cholesterol

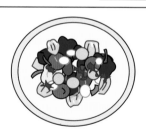

Monday's date _____

PHYSICAL ACTIVITY LOG

Record your physical activity for each day of the week. Older kids, record all of your physical activity. (Ex: Ran a mile with Dad. Rode my bike a block to Drew's house.) Younger kids, write at least one word to indicate your physical activity. (Ex: Soccer)

Monday:	
Tuesday:	
Wednesday:	
Thursday:	
Friday:	
Saturday:	
Sunday:	

TIME TRACKER (optional)
Color in a section for every 10 minutes of exercise you have completed each day. Goal: 1 hour of daily exercise.

HEALTHY FOOD 9-SQUARE
Make a smile face or place a sticker for every healthy food, found in this book, that you've eaten this week.

WRITER & ARTIST'S CORNER
Make a sketch or write down thoughts about your exercise or healthy eating this week. Possible topics include: goals, nature, and food.

M
T
W
H
F
S
S

DO A DUATHLON

Reason to Do a Duathlon "Twice as Much Fun" In a duathlon you can run and ride your bike.

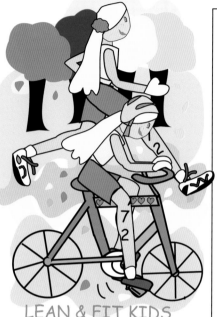

LEAN & FIT KIDS like to do more than one sport.

FUN FEET
Duathlon

Go for a run.

Take a drink of water.

Put on your helmet.

Get on your bike and go for a ride.

If you can, go for one more run.

PACK-A-SNACK
Baby Carrots

Eat plain.

Put in salads.

Eat with tofu dip

Add to soup.

Cook in stew.

Grate and add to muffins.

Bring to school.

GOOD STUFF
Carrots

-Lots of vitamin A to help your eyes

-Fiber

-Vitamin C

-Low in fat and no cholesterol

Monday's date _____

PHYSICAL ACTIVITY LOG

Record your physical activity for each day of the week. Older kids, record all of your physical activity. (Ex: Ran a mile with Dad. Rode my bike a block to Drew's house.) Younger kids, write at least one word to indicate your physical activity. (Ex: Soccer)

Monday:

Tuesday:

Wednesday:

Thursday:

Friday:

Saturday:

Sunday:

TIME TRACKER (optional)	HEALTHY FOOD 9-SQUARE	WRITER & ARTIST'S CORNER
Color in a section for every 10 minutes of exercise you have completed each day. Goal: 1 hour of daily exercise.	Make a smile face or place a sticker for every healthy food, found in this book, that you've eaten this week.	Make a sketch or write down thoughts about your exercise or healthy eating this week. Possible topics include: goals, nature, and food.

M
T
W
H
F
S
S

ADOPT A TREE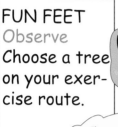

Reason to Adopt a Tree "Friendship" If you visit your tree often, it will become an old friend.

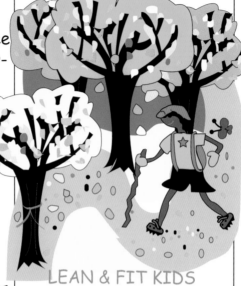

FUN FEET

Observe

Choose a tree on your exercise route.

Visit it at least once a week.

Sketch your tree.

Note changes.

LEAN & FIT KIDS

learn a lot about nature while they exercise.

PACK-A-SNACK

Healthy Oatmeal Cookies

1/3 c canola oil
3 Tbsp brown sugar
1 egg
1 tsp vanilla
3/4 c whole-wheat flour
1/2 tsp baking soda
1 1/2 c rolled oats
2 Tbsp raisins
1/4 c ground walnuts
1/2 tsp cinnamon

Preheat oven to 350°. Mix all ingredients together. Spray cookie sheet with non-fat spray. Bake about 12 minutes or until done.

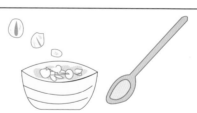

GOOD STUFF

Oatmeal
-Fiber

-Thiamine, magnesium, iron, and zinc

-A bowl of hot oatmeal (rolled oats) makes a great breakfast.

Monday's date _____

PHYSICAL ACTIVITY LOG

Record your physical activity for each day of the week. Older kids, record all of your physical activity. (Ex: Ran a mile with Dad. Rode my bike a block to Drew's house.) Younger kids, write at least one word to indicate your physical activity. (Ex: Soccer)

Monday:

Tuesday:

Wednesday:

Thursday:

Friday:

Saturday:

Sunday:

TIME TRACKER (optional)	HEALTHY FOOD 9-SQUARE	WRITER & ARTIST'S CORNER
Color in a section for every 10 minutes of exercise you have completed each day. Goal: 1 hour of daily exercise.	Make a smile face or place a sticker for every healthy food, found in this book, that you've eaten this week.	Make a sketch or write down thoughts about your exercise or healthy eating this week. Possible topics include: goals, nature, and food.

M
T
W
H
F
S
S

BIRDING

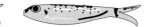

Reason to Go Birding "Wildlife" It's exciting to see differer types of birds in their natural habitats.

FUN FEET
Birding
Climb a tree to see a robin's nest.

Hike in a pine grove to spy a pileated woodpecker.

Jog on the shore and watch the seagulls fly.

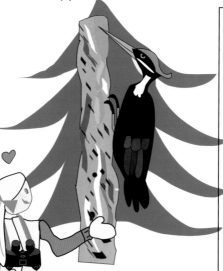

LEAN & FIT KIDS take long hikes which lead to new discoveries.

PACK-A-SNACK
Tiny Fish and Shellfish
Sardines on crackers with mustard

Anchovies in Caesar Salads

Oysters on toasted bread

It's easy to open little tins that hold tiny fish.

GOOD STUFF
Tiny Fish and Shellfish
-Omega-3 fats

-Protein

-Vitamin B$_{12}$

Omega-3 fats can help reduce bad cholesterol.
They can help your body make good cholesterol.
They can make your heart stay healthy.

Monday's date _____

PHYSICAL ACTIVITY LOG

Record your physical activity for each day of the week. Older kids, record all of your physical activity. (Ex: Ran a mile with Dad. Rode my bike a block to Drew's house.) Younger kids, write at least one word to indicate your physical activity. (Ex: Soccer)

Monday:

Tuesday:

Wednesday:

Thursday:

Friday:

Saturday:

Sunday:

TIME TRACKER (optional)	HEALTHY FOOD 9-SQUARE	WRITER & ARTIST'S CORNER
Color in a section for every 10 minutes of exercise you have completed each day. Goal: 1 hour of daily exercise.	Make a smile face or place a sticker for every healthy food, found in this book, that you've eaten this week.	Make a sketch or write down thoughts about your exercise or healthy eating this week. Possible topics include: goals, nature, and food.

M
T
W
H
F
S
S

DO MARTIAL ARTS

Reason to Do Martial Arts "In Shape" Practicing martial arts helps you keep in good shape.

FUN FEET
Martial Arts
Learn man-euvers for self defense.

Warm up with calis-thenics.

Learn flying kicks and punches.

Practice pro-tective blocks.

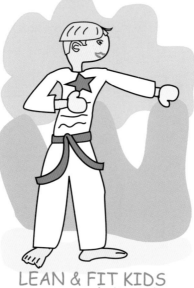

LEAN & FIT KIDS
use mental discipline to help stay in great physical condition.

PACK-A-SNACK
Soy Burgers
Try a flame broiled burger. Microwave and put on bun.

To make your burger even healthier, add lettuce, catsup, pickles, and tomatoes.

Eat it slowly and enjoy.

GOOD STUFF
Soy
-Protein

-Low in fat

-Low cholesterol

-Fiber

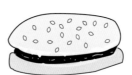

Soy is heart healthy.
Soy can reduce bad cholesterol.
Soy has healthy fat.
There are many different types of soy products.
You can enjoy soy for every meal, for snacks and for desserts.

Monday's date _____

PHYSICAL ACTIVITY LOG

Record your physical activity for each day of the week. Older kids, record all of your physical activity. (Ex: Ran a mile with Dad. Rode my bike a block to Drew's house.) Younger kids, write at least one word to indicate your physical activity. (Ex: Soccer)

Monday:

Tuesday:

Wednesday:

Thursday:

Friday:

Saturday:

Sunday:

TIME TRACKER (optional)
Color in a section for every 10 minutes of exercise you have completed each day. Goal: 1 hour of daily exercise.

HEALTHY FOOD 9-SQUARE
Make a smile face or place a sticker for every healthy food, found in this book, that you've eaten this week.

WRITER & ARTIST'S CORNER
Make a sketch or write down thoughts about your exercise or healthy eating this week. Possible topics include: goals, nature, and food.

M
T
W
T
F
S
S

NATURE HUNT

Reason to Nature Hunt "Treasures" You can find leaves that look like hearts, mittens, and stars.

FUN FEET
Nature Hunt

Catch a floating maple leaf.

Treasure a mitten-shaped sassafras leaf.

Hold a heart-shaped linden leaf.

Shine a light on a star-shaped sweetgum leaf.

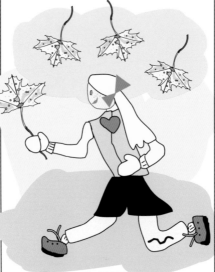

LEAN & FIT KIDS
enjoy physical activity so much that they often forget they are exercising.

PACK-A-SNACK
Burrito Egg Roll

1/2 c shredded red cabbage
1/2 c chopped red bell pepper
1/2 c chopped leeks
pinch of curry, tarragon, parsley, and salt
1 tsp olive oil
1/4 c Egg Beaters
1 whole-wheat wrap

Saute veggies until soft in olive oil. Add Egg Beaters and seasoning. Cook, stirring constantly until eggs are dry. Wrap and eat!

GOOD STUFF
Red Cabbage

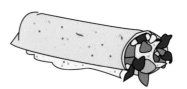

-Lots of vitamin C

-May protect against cancer

-Low in fat

-No cholesterol

Red cabbage looks almost purple when you buy it. It turns green when cooked in the Burrito Egg Roll recipe.

Monday's date _____

PHYSICAL ACTIVITY LOG

Record your physical activity for each day of the week. Older kids, record all of your physical activity. (Ex: Ran a mile with Dad. Rode my bike a block to Drew's house.) Younger kids, write at least one word to indicate your physical activity. (Ex: Soccer)

Monday:	
Tuesday:	
Wednesday:	
Thursday:	
Friday:	
Saturday:	
Sunday:	

TIME TRACKER (optional)	HEALTHY FOOD 9-SQUARE	WRITER & ARTIST'S CORNER
Color in a section for every 10 minutes of exercise you have completed each day. Goal: 1 hour of daily exercise.	Make a smile face or place a sticker for every healthy food, found in this book, that you've eaten this week.	Make a sketch or write down thoughts about your exercise or healthy eating this week. Possible topics include: goals, nature, and food.

M
T
W
H
F
S
S

HELP OTHERS
Reason to Help Others "Give Back" When you help others you make people happy.

FUN FEET
Give Back

Offer to shovel an elderly neighbor's walk.

Put on a "running" play for senior citizens.

Rake your grandparents' lawn.

Girl: I made some gingerbread cookies.
Boy: May I have one?
Girl: You may have one if you can run.
Boy: I can run.
Girl: But can you run fast?
Boy: I can run fast.
Girl: Then run fast! Run and catch my gingerbread girl.

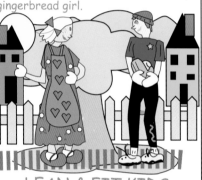

LEAN & FIT KIDS
use physical activity to do good deeds.

PACK-A-SNACK
Gingerbread Cookies
1/2 c dark molasses
1 egg
1 Tbsp milled flax seed
5 Tbsp canola oil
2 c whole-wheat pastry flour
1/2 tsp baking soda
1/4 tsp salt
1/2 tsp cinnamon and ginger
Preheat oven to 350°.
Prepare cookie sheet with no-fat spray. Mix. Roll dough 1/8-1/4 inch thick on floured board. Cut shapes with cookie cutters. Bake for about 10 minutes. These cookies are not very sweet, but they are healthy and delicious.

GOOD STUFF
Milled Flax Seed
-Fiber

-Omega-3 oils for healthy fat

-Whole grain

-No cholesterol

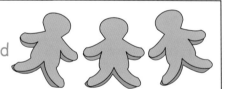

Monday's date _____

PHYSICAL ACTIVITY LOG

Record your physical activity for each day of the week. Older kids, record all of your physical activity. (Ex: Ran a mile with Dad. Rode my bike a block to Drew's house.) Younger kids, write at least one word to indicate your physical activity. (Ex: Soccer)

Monday:

Tuesday:

Wednesday:

Thursday:

Friday:

Saturday:

Sunday:

TIME TRACKER (optional)

Color in a section for every 10 minutes of exercise you have completed each day. Goal: 1 hour of daily exercise.

HEALTHY FOOD 9-SQUARE

Make a smile face or place a sticker for every healthy food, found in this book, that you've eaten this week.

WRITER & ARTIST'S CORNER

Make a sketch or write down thoughts about your exercise or healthy eating this week. Possible topics include: goals, nature, and food.

M
T
W
T
F
S
S

CANOE

Reason to Canoe "Explore" You can get to places that that you would never see without a canoe.

FUN FEET
Canoe
Paddle around a small pond.

Look at the plant life.

Search for ducks and turtles.

Enjoy the tranquility.

LEAN & FIT KIDS
feel great after a day of exercise.

PACK-A-SNACK
Papaya
Peel and eat.

Add to fruit salad, chicken salad, or seafood salad.

Buy or make papaya salsa.

Eat the black seeds, if you are brave. They taste peppery.

GOOD STUFF
Papaya

-Lots of vitamin C

-Low in fat

-No cholesterol

-Fiber

Monday's date _____

PHYSICAL ACTIVITY LOG

Record your physical activity for each day of the week. Older kids, record all of your physical activity. (Ex: Ran a mile with Dad. Rode my bike a block to Drew's house.) Younger kids, write at least one word to indicate your physical activity. (Ex: Soccer)

Monday:

Tuesday:

Wednesday:

Thursday:

Friday:

Saturday:

Sunday:

TIME TRACKER (optional)

Color in a section for every 10 minutes of exercise you have completed each day. Goal: 1 hour of daily exercise.

HEALTHY FOOD 9-SQUARE

Make a smile face or place a sticker for every healthy food, found in this book, that you've eaten this week.

WRITER & ARTIST'S CORNER

Make a sketch or write down thoughts about your exercise or healthy eating this week. Possible topics include: goals, nature, and food.

M
T
W
H
F
S
S

GO CAMPING

Reason to Go Camping

"Be Primitive" You can get away from modern technology while enjoying the planet Earth.

FUN FEET
Go Camping

Pitch your tent.

Hike on a nature trail.

Gather kindling for a fire.

Run and play ball.

Sing songs around a campfire.

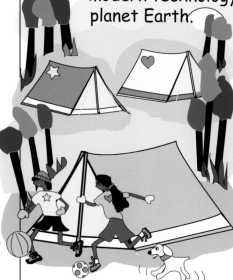

LEAN & FIT KIDS love to fall asleep in a sleeping bag after a fun-filled day in the wild.

PACK-A-SNACK
Chick Peas

Eat hummus with low-fat chips, whole-wheat bread, or raw veggies as a spread or dip.

Add to tuna, seafood, bean, or lettuce salads.

Heat and eat plain.

GOOD STUFF
Chick Peas

-Iron

-Fiber and Protein

-Low in fat

-No cholesterol

Monday's date _____

HYSICAL ACTIVITY LOG

ecord your physical activity for each day of the week. Older kids, record
ll of your physical activity. (Ex: Ran a mile with Dad. Rode my bike a block
o Drew's house.) Younger kids, write at least one word to indicate your
hysical activity. (Ex: Soccer)

Monday:

uesday:

Wednesday:

Thursday:

Friday:

Saturday:

Sunday:

TIME TRACKER (optional)	HEALTHY FOOD 9-SQUARE	WRITER & ARTIST'S CORNER
Color in a section for every 10 minutes of exercise you have completed each day. Goal: 1 hour of daily exercise.	Make a smile face or place a sticker for every healthy food, found in this book, that you've eaten this week.	Make a sketch or write down thoughts about your exercise or healthy eating this week. Possible topics include: goals, nature, and food.

M
T
W
H
F
S
S

RUN A 5-K

Reason to Run a 5-K

"Tradition" It's fun to choose a special 5-K to run every year with your family.

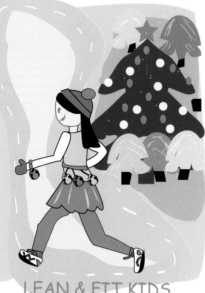

FUN FEET
5-K
Start training 6 weeks before a 5-K.

Run/walk short distances until you can run a mile or 2 each week.

Encourage yourself while you run. Think, "Easy does it! Doing great! Good job!"

LEAN & FIT KIDS
start out easy. They take walking breaks if they need them.

PACK-A-SNACK
Holiday Fruit Salad
1 red apple
1 green apple
1 yellow apple
1 peeled mango
1 peeled papaya
2 peeled kiwi
1 peeled banana
10 strawberries
10 maraschino cherries
1/4 c shredded coconut

Core apples, mango, and papaya. Cut all fruit into bite-sized pieces. Mix in a bowl. Sprinkle with coconut.

GOOD STUFF
Kiwi

-Lots of vitamin C

-No fat

-No cholesterol

-Fiber

Monday's date _____

PHYSICAL ACTIVITY LOG

Record your physical activity for each day of the week. Older kids, record all of your physical activity. (Ex: Ran a mile with Dad. Rode my bike a block to Drew's house.) Younger kids, write at least one word to indicate your physical activity. (Ex: Soccer)

| Monday: |
| Tuesday: |
| Wednesday: |
| Thursday: |
| Friday: |
| Saturday: |
| Sunday: |

TIME TRACKER (optional)
Color in a section for every 10 minutes of exercise you have completed each day. Goal: 1 hour of daily exercise.

HEALTHY FOOD 9-SQUARE
Make a smile face or place a sticker for every healthy food, found in this book, that you've eaten this week.

WRITER & ARTIST'S CORNER
Make a sketch or write down thoughts about your exercise or healthy eating this week. Possible topics include: goals, nature, and food.

M
T
W
H
F
S
S

FISH

Reason to Fish "Surprise" It's fun to feel a tug on your fishing line, but it's really exciting to see what's on your hook.

FUN FEET
Go Fishing

Catch a brook trout. It's too small, so throw it back.

Catch a catfish. It's big enough. Fill a bucket with pond water. Keep it fresh until supper time.

LEAN & FIT KIDS often choose fish as their source of protein.

PACK-A-SNACK
Salmon Salad

1/3 c cooked salmon (Canned or leftover salmon is great for this recipe.)
1/4 c chopped celery
2 tsp flavored light mayonnaise

Mix the salmon, celery, and mayonnaise.

Serve with reduced-fat Triscuit crackers.

GOOD STUFF
Salmon

-Omega-3 fish oil (heart and brain healthy)

-B vitamins (nervous system, blood, and brain healthy)

-Calcium (bone building) and protein (for growing)

-The fatty skin on the salmon is healthy.

Inspired by Payton, age 7, whose sister Cheyenne once caught a large mouth bass.

Monday's date _____

PHYSICAL ACTIVITY LOG

Record your physical activity for each day of the week. Older kids, record all of your physical activity. (Ex: Ran a mile with Dad. Rode my bike a block to Drew's house.) Younger kids, write at least one word to indicate your physical activity. (Ex: Soccer)

Monday:

Tuesday:

Wednesday:

Thursday:

Friday:

Saturday:

Sunday:

TIME TRACKER (optional)	HEALTHY FOOD 9-SQUARE	WRITER & ARTIST'S CORNER
Color in a section for every 10 minutes of exercise you have completed each day. Goal: 1 hour of daily exercise.	Make a smile face or place a sticker for every healthy food, found in this book, that you've eaten this week.	Make a sketch or write down thoughts about your exercise or healthy eating this week. Possible topics include: goals, nature, and food.

M
T
W
TH
F
S
S

Revisit a Route
Reason to Revisit a Route "Heaven on Earth" A special runnir route can make you feel happy.

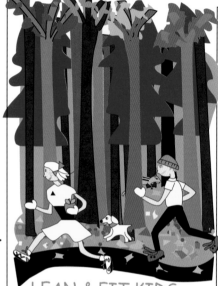

FUN FEET
Your Route
Find a route with lots of tall trees.

See its busy squirrels and chipmunks.

Listen to its babbling brook.

Return to your route whenever you can.

LEAN & FIT KIDS
have a place outdoors which feels like home.

PACK-A-SNACK
Cantaloupe
Eat plain.

Add to fruit salads.

Eat with breakfast, lunch, or dinner.

Cut into chunks and take to school for a healthy snack.

GOOD STUFF
Cantaloupe
-Vitamin A for healthy skin

-Vitamin C to promote healing of wounds

-Low in calories

-Beta carotene to protect against disease

Monday's date _____

PHYSICAL ACTIVITY LOG

Record your physical activity for each day of the week. Older kids, record all of your physical activity. (Ex: Ran a mile with Dad. Rode my bike a block to Drew's house.) Younger kids, write at least one word to indicate your physical activity. (Ex: Soccer)

Monday:

Tuesday:

Wednesday:

Thursday:

Friday:

Saturday:

Sunday:

TIME TRACKER (optional)	HEALTHY FOOD 9-SQUARE	WRITER & ARTIST'S CORNER
Color in a section for every 10 minutes of exercise you have completed each day. Goal: 1 hour of daily exercise.	Make a smile face or place a sticker for every healthy food, found in this book, that you've eaten this week.	Make a sketch or write down thoughts about your exercise or healthy eating this week. Possible topics include: goals, nature, and food.

RIDE A HORSE
Reason to Ride a Horse "Confidence" Learning to ride and handle a horse can increase your confidence.

FUN FEET
Ride a Horse

Ride a pony in a corral.

Spend some time grooming a horse.

Walk a horse on a trail.

Go a little faster. Tell your horse to trot.

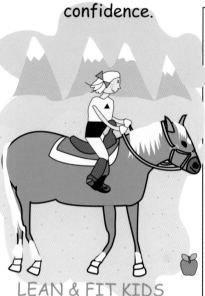

LEAN & FIT KIDS
enjoy activities which increase their muscle strength and balance.

PACK-A-SNACK
Sweet Corn

Corn on the cob

Corn kernels

Salsa with corn

Corn pudding

Corn chowder

Cornmeal muffins

Corn chutney

GOOD STUFF
Corn

-Fiber

-Low in fat

-Vitamin C

-Vitamin B1

Monday's date _____

PHYSICAL ACTIVITY LOG

Record your physical activity for each day of the week. Older kids, record all of your physical activity. (Ex: Ran a mile with Dad. Rode my bike a block to Drew's house.) Younger kids, write at least one word to indicate your physical activity. (Ex: Soccer)

Monday:
Tuesday:
Wednesday:
Thursday:
Friday:
Saturday:
Sunday:

TIME TRACKER (optional)

Color in a section for every 10 minutes of exercise you have completed each day. Goal: 1 hour of daily exercise.

HEALTHY FOOD 9-SQUARE

Make a smile face or place a sticker for every healthy food, found in this book, that you've eaten this week.

WRITER & ARTIST'S CORNER

Make a sketch or write down thoughts about your exercise or healthy eating this week. Possible topics include: goals, nature, and food.

RAKE LEAVES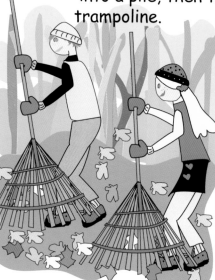

Reason to Rake Leaves

"Leaf Pile" You can rake leaves into a pile, then treat it like a trampoline.

FUN FEET
Rake Leaves

Rake the leaves in your back yard.

Make a pile.

Play a little - run and jump.

Roll around.

Then rake some more.

LEAN & FIT KIDS can find lots of ways to stay active at home.

PACK-A-SNACK
Celery

Add to tuna or egg salad.

Use in chicken soup.

Fill with healthy peanut butter. Sprinkle with raisins.

Add to bread stuffing.

GOOD STUFF
Celery

-Low in fat and calories

-Fiber

-Gives crunch and great taste to lots of healthy foods

Monday's date _____

PHYSICAL ACTIVITY LOG

Record your physical activity for each day of the week. Older kids, record all of your physical activity. (Ex: Ran a mile with Dad. Rode my bike a block to Drew's house.) Younger kids, write at least one word to indicate your physical activity. (Ex: Soccer)

Monday:

Tuesday:

Wednesday:

Thursday:

Friday:

Saturday:

Sunday:

TIME TRACKER (optional)	HEALTHY FOOD 9-SQUARE	WRITER & ARTIST'S CORNER
Color in a section for every 10 minutes of exercise you have completed each day. Goal: 1 hour of daily exercise.	Make a smile face or place a sticker for every healthy food, found in this book, that you've eaten this week.	Make a sketch or write down thoughts about your exercise or healthy eating this week. Possible topics include: goals, nature, and food.

GARDEN
Reason to Garden "Delicious Food" Vegetables taste better fresh from the garden.

FUN FEET
Garden
Work the soil.

Rake and hoe.

Build a fence.

Plant your seeds.

Water and weed.

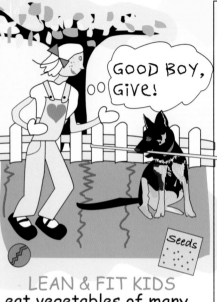

GOOD BOY, GIVE!

LEAN & FIT KIDS
eat vegetables of many colors.

Seeds

PACK-A-SNACK
Green Beans
Trim and eat fresh. Pack with carrots, and red peppers for a colorful snack.

Add to tuna, egg, or garden salad.

Cook and eat with lunch or supper.

GOOD STUFF
Green Beans
-Low in fat and lots of fiber

-Vitamin C

-It's educational to watch green beans grow, because the cotyledons emerge from the seed coat above the ground.

Monday's date _____

PHYSICAL ACTIVITY LOG

Record your physical activity for each day of the week. Older kids, record all of your physical activity. (Ex: Ran a mile with Dad. Rode my bike a block to Drew's house.) Younger kids, write at least one word to indicate your physical activity. (Ex: Soccer)

Monday:
Tuesday:
Wednesday:
Thursday:
Friday:
Saturday:
Sunday:

TIME TRACKER (optional)

Color in a section for every 10 minutes of exercise you have completed each day. Goal: 1 hour of daily exercise.

M
T
W
H
F
S
S

HEALTHY FOOD 9-SQUARE

Make a smile face or place a sticker for every healthy food, found in this book, that you've eaten this week.

WRITER & ARTIST'S CORNER

Make a sketch or write down thoughts about your exercise or healthy eating this week. Possible topics include: goals, nature, and food.

HURDLE
Reason to Hurdle
"Soaring" Jumping over obstacles while on a run makes you feel like an eagle.

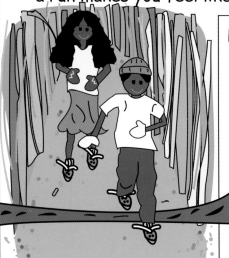

FUN FEET
Hurdle

Jump over a few logs.

Hurdle fallen branches.

Spring in and out of old tires.

Play leap frog.

LEAN & FIT KIDS
love to leap over things.

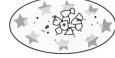

PACK-A-SNACK
Pesto Sauce

2 Tbsp extra virgin olive oil
1 Tbsp grated sharp Italian cheese (or Parmesan cheese)
1 clove garlic
pinch of basil, parsley flakes, and thyme
2 large walnut pieces

Put into blender and blend at medium speed.

Use as pasta sauce, bread dip, or drizzle over a garden salad. Serves 4.

GOOD STUFF
Olive Oil

-Good fat which lowers "bad" cholesterol

-Choose "extra-virgin" olive oil.

-Olive oil is good for you, but high in calories, so watch your portion size.

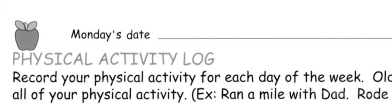

Monday's date _____

PHYSICAL ACTIVITY LOG

Record your physical activity for each day of the week. Older kids, record all of your physical activity. (Ex: Ran a mile with Dad. Rode my bike a block to Drew's house.) Younger kids, write at least one word to indicate your physical activity. (Ex: Soccer)

Monday:
Tuesday:
Wednesday:
Thursday:
Friday:
Saturday:
Sunday:

TIME TRACKER (optional)

Color in a section for every 10 minutes of exercise you have completed each day. Goal: 1 hour of daily exercise.

M
T
W
H
F
S
S

HEALTHY FOOD 9-SQUARE

Make a smile face or place a sticker for every healthy food, found in this book, that you've eaten this week.

WRITER & ARTIST'S CORNER

Make a sketch or write down thoughts about your exercise or healthy eating this week. Possible topics include: goals, nature, and food.

DO A TRIATHLON

Reason to Do a Triathlon "Three Times as Much Fun" In a
triathlon you swim, run, and cycle.

FUN FEET
Triathlon

Have your
own fun
triathlon.

Go for a swim
in a pool or
pond.

Jump on your
bike and ride.

Finish up with
a little run.

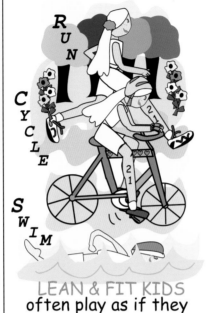

LEAN & FIT KIDS
often play as if they
were in a real event.

PACK-A-SNACK
Cranberry Relish

12 ounce package fresh
cranberries
2 medium or 1 large orange
1/2 c frozen raspberries
3 Tbsp sugar
1 Tbsp honey

Rinse cranberries.
Peel orange(s) and
remove seeds. Blend
ingredients in blender
or food processor.

Eat as is, or eat
with crackers,
cottage cheese,
fruit, or veggies.

GOOD STUFF
Cranberries

-Low in fat and calories

-Vitamin C

-Cranberry relish goes great with a
turkey dinner.

Monday's date _____

PHYSICAL ACTIVITY LOG

Record your physical activity for each day of the week. Older kids, record all of your physical activity. (Ex: Ran a mile with Dad. Rode my bike a block to Drew's house.) Younger kids, write at least one word to indicate your physical activity. (Ex: Soccer)

Monday:
Tuesday:
Wednesday:
Thursday:
Friday:
Saturday:
Sunday:

TIME TRACKER (optional)

Color in a section for every 10 minutes of exercise you have completed each day. Goal: 1 hour of daily exercise.

HEALTHY FOOD 9-SQUARE

Make a smile face or place a sticker for every healthy food, found in this book, that you've eaten this week.

WRITER & ARTIST'S CORNER

Make a sketch or write down thoughts about your exercise or healthy eating this week. Possible topics include: goals, nature, and food.

M
T
W
H
F
S
S

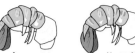

RUN A MILE
Reason to Run a Mile

"Popular Measure" The mile is a standard distance that you'll run in gym class and at fun runs.

FUN FEET
Run a Mile

Build gradually to the mile.

Run a 1/4 mile, then 1/2 mile.

Walk a mile.

Mix up your walking with some jogging.

Ready, set, go!

Run a mile.

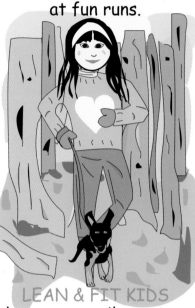

LEAN & FIT KIDS know many mile routes in their neighborhoods.

PACK-A-SNACK
Shrimp

Eat with cock-tail sauce.

Mix with light mayonnaise and celery for shrimp salad.

Add to a garden salad.

Make a shrimp omelet.

GOOD STUFF
Shrimp

-Low in fat

-Low in calories

-Omega-3 fatty acids

-Protein

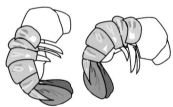

This page was inspired by Beatrice, age 7, who was born in China and loves to run.

Monday's date _____

PHYSICAL ACTIVITY LOG

Record your physical activity for each day of the week. Older kids, record all of your physical activity. (Ex: Ran a mile with Dad. Rode my bike a block to Drew's house.) Younger kids, write at least one word to indicate your physical activity. (Ex: Soccer)

Monday:

Tuesday:

Wednesday:

Thursday:

Friday:

Saturday:

Sunday:

TIME TRACKER (optional)	HEALTHY FOOD 9-SQUARE	WRITER & ARTIST'S CORNER
Color in a section for every 10 minutes of exercise you have completed each day. Goal: 1 hour of daily exercise.	Make a smile face or place a sticker for every healthy food, found in this book, that you've eaten this week.	Make a sketch or write down thoughts about your exercise or healthy eating this week. Possible topics include: goals, nature, and food.

M
T
W
H
F
S
S

STREGH

Reason to Stretch "Flexibility" Stretching before and after physical activity makes your muscles more pliable.

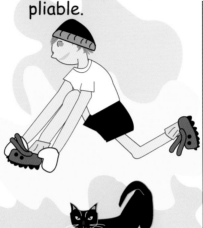

FUN FEET
Stretch
Jog to warm up.

Stretch your muscles from head to toe.

Exercise.

Stretch again when your exercise ends.

LEAN & FIT KIDS
stretch slowly without bouncing.

PACK-A-SNACK
Chocolate Chip Cookies
1 c plus 2 Tbsp whole-wheat pastry flour
3 Tbsp toasted wheat germ
1/2 tsp baking soda
1/2 tsp salt
1/3 c canola oil
1 egg
1 tsp vanilla
3 Tbsp brown sugar
3 Tbsp white sugar
1/3 c semi-sweet chocolate chips

Preheat oven to 350°. Prepare cookie sheet with Pam. Mix all ingredients. Use your hands to form dough into balls. Bake for 12 minutes or until done. Cool on wire rack.

GOOD STUFF

Wheat Germ
-Folic acid to help with red blood cell production

-Vitamin E which may help prevent cancer

-No cholesterol

Monday's date _____

PHYSICAL ACTIVITY LOG

Record your physical activity for each day of the week. Older kids, record all of your physical activity. (Ex: Ran a mile with Dad. Rode my bike a block to Drew's house.) Younger kids, write at least one word to indicate your physical activity. (Ex: Soccer)

Monday:

Tuesday:

Wednesday:

Thursday:

Friday:

Saturday:

Sunday:

TIME TRACKER (optional)	HEALTHY FOOD 9-SQUARE	WRITER & ARTIST'S CORNER
Color in a section for every 10 minutes of exercise you have completed each day. Goal: 1 hour of daily exercise.	Make a smile face or place a sticker for every healthy food, found in this book, that you've eaten this week.	Make a sketch or write down thoughts about your exercise or healthy eating this week. Possible topics include: goals, nature, and food.

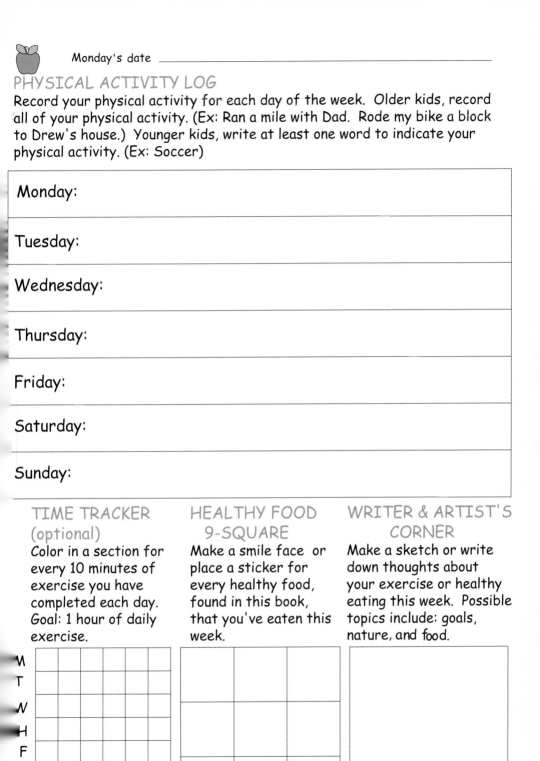

RUN
Reason to Run

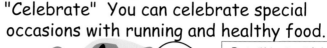

"Celebrate" You can celebrate special occasions with running and healthy food.

FUN FEET
Run

Go for a long run on the first day of spring.

Run a fun run with Mom on Mother's Day.

Create a birthday obstacle course for your friends.

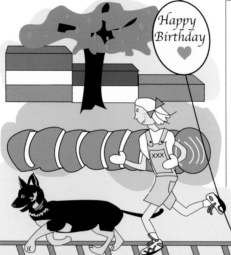

Happy Birthday ♥

PACK-A-SNACK
Cherries

Fill and top your birthday cake with light (no sugar) cherry pie filling, instead of frosting.

Serve with a smoothie made from non-fat yogurt, cherries, kiwi, oranges, strawberries and orange juice.

LEAN & FIT KIDS
want to participate in their favorite physical activities on their birthdays.

GOOD STUFF
Cherries
-Vitamin C

-Vitamin A

-No cholesterol

-Fiber

Monday's date _____

HYSICAL ACTIVITY LOG

ecord your physical activity for each day of the week. Older kids, record
ll of your physical activity. (Ex: Ran a mile with Dad. Rode my bike a block
o Drew's house.) Younger kids, write at least one word to indicate your
hysical activity. (Ex: Soccer)

Monday:

uesday:

Vednesday:

hursday:

riday:

Saturday:

unday:

TIME TRACKER
(optional)
Color in a section for
every 10 minutes of
exercise you have
completed each day.
Goal: 1 hour of daily
exercise.

HEALTHY FOOD
9-SQUARE
Make a smile face or
place a sticker for
every healthy food,
found in this book,
that you've eaten this
week.

WRITER & ARTIST'S
CORNER
Make a sketch or write
down thoughts about
your exercise or healthy
eating this week. Possible
topics include: goals,
nature, and food.

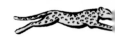
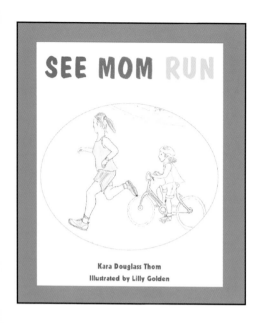
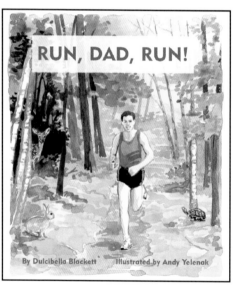
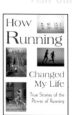
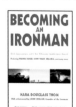
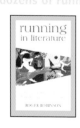
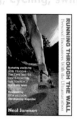
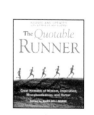
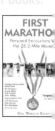